The Biomedical Sciences in Society

Iain Crinson

The Biomedical Sciences in Society

An Interdisciplinary Analysis

palgrave
macmillan

Iain Crinson
St Georges
University of London
London, UK

ISBN 978-981-15-9522-6 ISBN 978-981-15-9523-3 (eBook)
https://doi.org/10.1007/978-981-15-9523-3

This Palgrave Macmillan imprint is published by the registered company Springer Nature Singapore Pte Ltd.
The registered company address is: 152 Beach Road, #21-01/04 Gateway East, Singapore 189721, Singapore

Contents

Contents

List of Figures

List of Tables

The Interdisciplinarity Field of Social Studies of Science and Technology (SSST)

1

Abstract

This chapter provides a general introduction to the main themes of the book. It then moves on to an introductory discussion of interdisciplinarity, which is now a mainstream approach to research and analysis in both the social and natural sciences. It focuses in particular on the movement towards interdisciplinary within the biomedical sciences. This is followed by an account of the historical emergence of increasing social and political concerns about the uses and abuses of scientific knowledge and innovative technologies that led eventually to the establishment of the academic field of Social Studies of Science and Technology (SSST). A series of examples are then provided to illustrate the scope of this field.

General Introduction

Over the course of the last three decades, the research horizons of biomedical science have widened to such an extent that the disciplinary boundaries that once clearly demarcated the scope of knowledge of the social and the natural worlds have begun to crumble. The promissory visions set out in the research programmes of biomedical science increasingly involve pushing the frontiers of scientific knowledge generation beyond the threshold of the human body and into the domain of the social. For example, recent developments in both the neurosciences and genomics now offer radically new ways to re-imagine a range of contemporary social concerns through the lens of neural pathways or epigenetic modifications. Nevertheless, alongside these 'out of the lab' initiatives have emerged new and frequently unanticipated social, bioethical, and legal dilemmas and challenges.

The aim of this textbook is to provide a comprehensive introduction to a wide range of social analysis that has sought to assess and contextualise this expanding role for the biomedical sciences. The research cited in this book therefore ranges

I. Crinson, *The Biomedical Sciences in Society*,
https://doi.org/10.1007/978-981-15-9523-3_1

from micro-level studies of interactions between scientists in the laboratory as they seek to further their understanding of microbiological processes through to a macro-level analysis of the decision-making processes involved in the construction of regulatory frameworks for the governance of biomedical research. From questions about the level of trust that the public place in expert knowledge and scientific innovation to concerns about the commercial exploitation of personal biomaterial altruistically donated to biobanks. There is a critical assessment of why colour-coded brain scans used to represent the workings of the human brain have such an 'allure' for the media and the public and a detailed examination of the challenges faced in delivering on the promise of a pharmacogenomic-based system of disease management. These and many other areas of social analysis and research, which are focused on the impact of biomedical science in society, together constitute the interdisciplinary (ITD) field known as Social Studies of Science and Technology (SSST).

A key objective of this textbook is to describe and demonstrate the analytical tools drawn upon within SSST in order to enable the reader to develop their own informed and critical assessment of the role now played by the biomedical sciences in the social world. A second objective is to make a contribution to building a mutual understanding and constructive dialogue between the social and biomedical sciences. Such an engagement can only enhance future interdisciplinary work that addresses, for example, the common health challenges now faced by societies across the globe.

Who Is This Textbook Intended for?

The intended primary readership for this textbook are final-year undergraduate and post-graduates studying 'science in society' type modules that are increasingly being included within social, political, or biomedical science academic programmes of study. The material in this book can also be utilised as a primer for those intending to undertake post-graduate research, particularly if engaged in boundary work between the social and biological worlds. The text is constructed so as to enable those with limited biomedical science knowledge to get to grips with the major developments within the field and for those with a limited working knowledge of the social sciences to gain an understanding of the key social theoretical and conceptual approaches that are drawn upon when contextualising the dynamic interrelationship between biomedicine and society.

There has also been a significant upsurge in the public interest in developments within the biomedical sciences, not least in terms of the social impact of pandemics such as Covid-19 and the public trust afforded to expert knowledge. This book is therefore also designed to be accessible to an informed general readership interested in a wide-ranging analysis of these developments as they impact on social life.

Interdisciplinarity in Research and Analysis

Over the last three decades or so, the requirement for academic research to bridge the traditional disciplinary boundaries of science has been widely recognised. Today, the prevailing view is that interdisciplinary (ITD) research is the most appropriate strategy for advancing the knowledge and technological innovations that are capable of addressing new and ever more demanding societal, environmental, and industrial challenges. ITD research has therefore come to be 'at once a governmental demand, a reflexive orientation within the academy, and an object of knowledge' (Barry and Born 2013: 4). Yet it is difficult to provide an unambiguous definition of ITD. It is perhaps best understood as an umbrella or generic term that draws attention to a multiplicity of intellectual practices involving the coming together of disciplinary knowledge applied to specific real-world problems. Today, examples of ITD research practice can be found across both the natural and the social sciences, and increasingly the arts and humanities too. In 2015, the prestigious science journal *Nature* published a special issue (Volume 525) in support of the view that ITD was 'considered crucial' for the future of scientific development. One of the papers included in this special issue drew upon an analysis of the Web of Science database, involving 14 major academic disciplines and 143 sub-specialities. The report concluded that since the mid-1980s, research papers in both the social and natural sciences have increasingly cited work outside their own disciplines, with the field of health and biosciences research found to be the most interdisciplinary of all (Van Noorden 2015).

ITD research practice involves engaging in a process of synthesis, subsuming disciplinary-based theories and concepts to meet specific research goals. But this process should also be a reflexive one that involves a mutual appreciation of both the strengths and limitations that each disciplinary perspective brings to a common research objective. The limitations of a single disciplinary-based approach can involve a tendency towards the promotion of orthodoxy, 'carving up the universe of intellectual problems into minute and meaningless increments' (Jasanoff 2013: 99). While the strengths lie in the conceptual depth and established models of causality found in single disciplines, so 'that without disciplines, interdisciplinarity would be inconceivable' (Mäki 2016: 331).

The literature identifies a range of imperatives for promoting ITD approaches to research and analysis. One key driver of ITD being the necessity of breaking down the barriers that have traditionally problematised the relationship between science and the society, particularly in terms of public trust. The adoption of ITD research is often presented as leading onto a re-orientation of the institutional practices of research organisations, enabling them to break free from their esoteric and introspective boundaries and interests, to engage in open 'knowledge dialogues' with the public. A second driver is the increasing requirement for publically funded science research to respond more proactively to the social and economic needs of a society. A third and decisive driver is the belated recognition that the inherent complexity and uncertainty of the world are not easily captured within traditional single disciplinary research methodologies. Recognising the necessity for ITD approaches is an acknowledgment that new methodologies are required to address unanticipated challenges arising from the interplay of multiple and irreducible natural and social mechanisms (Bhaskar Danermark and Price 2018: 27).

Relatively recent developments in both national and supra-national research strategy and funding have played an important role in promoting the shift towards ITD. A prominent example would be the European Union's 'Horizon 2020' research and innovation programme, funded to the tune of some €80 billion over a seven-year period from 2014 to 2020. A key working principle of H2020 has been to 'stimulate a breakdown of the silos of different research disciplines and stimulate integration in order to maximize impact' (EU 2014). Of the €80 billion total research budget, €28 billion was specifically allocated to meeting 'societal challenges'. This objective necessitated new levels of cooperation and integration between disciplinary fields in both the natural and social sciences (Allmendinger 2015). The European Research Council (ERC), and many national research funding organisations, now explicitly promotes and facilitates ITD research projects. While in the UK, the Higher Education Academy and the Research Councils have long sought to promote ITD in both teaching and research. In 2018, the largely single disciplinary-based research councils were re-organised and centralised and became UK Research and Innovation (UKRI). This quasi-autonomous umbrella body was established through primary legislation to effectively manage the government's science budget (see also Chap. 9). It now manages 'cross-council funding' programmes which include the promotion of 'interdisciplinary research hubs' to address new global and social challenges (www.ukri.org). The Human Genome Project (HGP) would be one outstanding example of a successful interdisciplinary biomedical science research programme, the outcomes of which continue to have a profound impact on medicine and science in society. Today, the intellectual and research practices associated with ITD research science are sufficiently well established that they themselves have become an object of academic research and evaluation, under the heading of 'Interdisciplinary Studies'.

Interdisciplinarity in the Biomedical Sciences

Interdisciplinarity has always been a characteristic feature of the biomedical sciences. The history of one of its core disciplines, biology, is one that has been shaped by its interaction with other disciplines over the centuries. Biology and chemistry first came together in the mid-nineteenth century, combining to conduct the first studies of organic molecules and their chemical reactions within living systems. Biologists began working with mathematicians in the early twentieth century in order to study disease transmission patterns in populations. During the mid-twentieth century, biologists working with engineers developed some of the first medical devices such as heart pace-makers, and later still diagnostic imaging machines (together with physicists). More recently, bioengineers have furthered the understanding of how mechanical forces operate at the molecular level, for example, in the walls of the heart to help regulate cardiac growth during normal development and in disease states (Burggren et al. 2017: 106).

The biological study of the natural world has long been intertwined with the practice of medicine. In Ancient Greece, some 2400 years ago, Aristotle's observations of living animals, combined with his dissections and experiments, were used to advance an understanding of the anatomy, physiology, and pathology of various animal species. Earlier still, in the fifth-century BC, Hippocrates and his followers, 'elevated themselves above root-gatherers, diviners and others whom they dismissed as ignoramuses and quacks … (and) promoted *natural* theories of health and sickness grounded upon superior *natural* knowledge, and *natural* modes of healing' (Porter 2003: 25—emphasis in original). Hippocrates' close observations sought to understand health and illness in terms of the changing rhythms of key bodily fluids ('humours'). An imbalance between these fluids (blood, phlegm, yellow bile, and black bile) was seen to result in illness, but this could be corrected through diet or other interventions such as blood-letting. This approach known as 'humouralism' went onto define the classical medical approach for centuries, noting that this holistic approach to healing was also the basis of the Ayurvedic system of medicine practised in the Indian sub-continent from ancient times. This tradition of health as defined by biological homeostasis was enhanced by its adoption within the system of Galenic medicine emergent in the second-century Roman Empire. However, it eventually succumbed to the advances made in the understanding of human physiology (dissection had been explicitly forbidden in Ancient Greece) achieved in the 'Golden Age' of Islamic medicine in the twelfth and thirteenth centuries. One example would be the work of Ibn al-Nafis, an Arab physician who made important advances in the early knowledge of the pulmonary circulation. The contribution of Islamic medicine was crucial to the later developments in human biology that occurred in Renaissance Europe in the sixteenth century. This marked the early beginnings of what was to become known as the 'Age of Enlightenment', the root of modern science. Nonetheless, it was the early Greek understanding of holism that firmly established the interconnectivity between, 'the natural and the human, the physical and the mental, the healthy and the pathological' (Porter 2003: 30). That is, if we read 'the natural' as the biological, the close observation of signs and symptoms as 'scientific method', and for the profession of healing we read 'the practice of medicine'.

The history of medicine is not one in which knowledge and practice progresses systematically and accumulates over time; it has been very much a stop-start process, and in some cases 'one step forward, two steps backward'. For example, William Harvey's revolutionary research into the circulation of blood through the heart at the beginning of the seventeenth century was the first major development in the understanding of blood flow for nearly 400 years. But from the late eighteenth century onwards, the opening of new hospitals to provide shelter and support for the sick deserving poor in the expanding urban centres of Western Europe offered the opportunity to undertake the first systematic close observations of illnesses. The incipient studies of human disease that followed in the early to mid-nineteenth century 'leveraged our knowledge and understanding of health, and vice versa'

(Burggren et al. 2017: 103). Louis Pasteur's careful experimental work in the 1880s (he was a chemist by training) was the first to demonstrate that it was microbes that were the cause of infectious disease. It was Pasteur's linking of streptococci and staphylococci to specific diseases that introduced bacteriology into the practice of medicine. By the beginning of the twentieth century, a new academic field of biological chemistry was being integrated into the pre-clinical curricula of US medical schools, then going through a dramatic structural development. These reforms to the training of doctors reflected an increasing understanding that basic biological knowledge and methods were crucial to the development of a modern medicine (Kohler 1982: 6).

Over the course of the twentieth century, other scientific disciplines, such as psychology, physics, engineering, and latterly informatics, have come to play a role not only in medical education, but also in the dramatic expansion of the research boundaries of biomedical science. It was the merger of molecular biology and genetics to establish the field of genomics (the study of genes and their functions) at the close of the last century that enabled medicine, 'to address the questions of health and disease as a continuum (rather than singular pathological events per se), based on genetic mechanisms as they apply to the relevant phenotypes' (Burggren et al. 2017: 103—comment in parenthesis not in original).

Social Studies of Scientific Knowledge (SSK)

A new field of social research and analysis emerged in the late 1960s, one that reflected a growing set of social and political concerns about the uses and abuses of scientific knowledge and innovative technologies. This was a historical period that was witnessing the first mass promotion of pharmaceuticals to alleviate social stresses and anxiety, for example, Diazepam ('Valium'); the intensification of agriculture with the use of chemical pesticides on a global scale; the uninhibited construction of nuclear power plants for the production of 'clean' energy, not to mention weapons grade plutonium; the exploration of space and the use of satellite technologies not only for global communication but also for military surveillance; and the proliferation of weapons of biological warfare, notably in the form of 'Agent Orange' that was extensively utilised by the US Air force in their bombing campaigns in Vietnam and Cambodia in the late 1960s. It was their involvement in the student protests against the Vietnam war, in both Europe and North America, that prompted concerned groups of young scientists to set up associations such as Scientists and Engineers for Social and Political Action (SESPA) in the USA and the British Society for Social Responsibility of Science (BSSRS). It was these organisations that were behind the early drive for the establishment of interdisciplinary social research programmes to more closely analyse and monitor the sources of funding and the social impact and direction of science.

One of the key intellectual stumbling blocks in this new field of research was the question of what intellectual tools should be applied in establishing a critical analysis of the role of science in society? In 1962, Thomas Kuhn had published his book,

'*The Structure of Scientific Revolutions*', which had an immediate impact in challenging some of the key shibboleths of scientific work (discussed in detail in Chap. 2). Kuhn's thesis was that the history of science as one marked by a steady cumulative progress in understanding the natural world was essentially a myth. His conclusion was that science, far from operating through stable and established methods, was actually characterised by 'alternating "normal" and "revolutionary" phases, in which communities of specialists are plunged into periods of turmoil and uncertainty … this understanding posed a challenge to powerful, entrenched philosophical assumptions about how science did, and should work' (Naughton 2012). Kuhn was not a philosopher by training (he was in fact a physicist), but his theoretical work rested on a close reading of historical studies of science. Yet however insightful his conclusions were, his methodology was not one that could be easily repurposed to construct a social scientific critique of science knowledge. However, inspiration was found in the methodology being advanced by two sociologists, Berger and Luckmann, in their book, '*The Social Construction of Reality: A Treatise in the Sociology of Knowledge*', first published in 1966.

Berger and Luckmann (1967) defined their theoretical focus as '(W)hatever passes for knowledge in a society regardless of the ultimate validity or invalidity (by whatever criteria) of such "knowledge". And in so far as all human knowledge is developed, transmitted and maintained in social situations, the sociology of knowledge must seek to understand the processes by which this is done in such a way that a taken-for-granted reality congeals for the man in the street' (1967: 17). Berger and Luckmann went onto assert that we come to know the world we inhabit through the ideas and beliefs we hold about it, so that it is our concepts and categories that become the realities of the world for us. This is not to deny the existence of objective realities, but simply a recognition that our understanding of these realities is always mediated by our subjective interpretations. In turn, these interpretations are seen as shaped by a wide range of social processes and institutions. Although Berger and Luckmann's work was concerned with how knowledge is constructed and directed towards resolving the practical problems of everyday life, their 'social constructionist' approach was soon to be applied by others in relation to formalised scientific knowledge.

The first and most notable example of the insistence that science could not, and should not, be exempt from sociological analysis was the establishment of the research programme known as the 'Sociology of Scientific Knowledge', which was instigated at Edinburgh University in the early 1970s. David Bloor and Barry Barnes were two of the key figures in the decision that was made to adopt an 'anti-realist' (this philosophical principle is discussed in detail in Chap. 2) frame of analysis for the SSK programme. As such, the focus of academic activity was not philosophical debate per se, but a critical engagement with the various truth claims of science. This approach drew upon a naturalist methodological approach that privileged the researchers own observations, descriptions, and interpretations of the experiences and actions of specific groups of scientists within a socio-cultural context. For Bloor, naturalistic methods require that, '(A)ll knowledge, whether it be in the empirical sciences or even in mathematics, should be treated, through and through, as material for investigation' (Bloor 1991: 1). The SSK programme set itself the task of demonstrating that the developments within science and technology should be framed by the study of the actual practice of scientists and engineers as an object of empirical investigation, in and of itself. As such, SSK became associated with what has been termed the 'strong version' of social constructionist analysis. The latter references natural objects conceived only as referents of scientific knowledge, and therefore entirely socially contingent.

SSK as a field of analysis was subsequently to be riven the so-called 'science wars' of the early 1990s. These cultural debates revolved around the determination of a number of well-known natural scientists to undermine the key premises of SSK and to challenge its authority as a social institution capable of realising truths about the scientific world. The critics (which included the mathematician Norman Levitt, the biologist Paul Gross, and the physicist Alan Sokal) asserted that social theory alone was inadequate to the task of analysing 'objective science'. This was a criticism that was subsequently to be accepted by several key figures within the SSK camp, including Bruno Latour and John Law, who both now acknowledged that there could be no place outside of nature or the socio-cultural where a purely objective study of science could place itself. Already by the late 1980s, Latour had suggested that 'social sciences are part of the problem, not of the solution' (Latour 1988: 161). Dissenting voices in SSK, including Latour's, went onto develop a very different approach to the study of science and technology, one that sought to go beyond the perceived limitations of 'the social' as applying only to human agency. This approach subsequently became known as 'Actor Network Theory' (ANT)—(see Theory Box 3.1 in Chap. 3).

The 'Discipline' of Science and Technology Studies (STS)

SSST is the umbrella term utilised throughout this textbook to denote the interdisciplinary field of research and analysis of science and technology in society. This field embraces a wide range of social science and humanities-based disciplinary studies, accompanied by their distinct modes of analysis and perspective (a scenario is set out in the final section of this chapter to demonstrate these differences). Situated within, but also at the same time outside this field of interdisciplinary analysis, is a singular approach to studying science in society, known as Science and Technology Studies (STS). These studies have made a valuable contribution to furthering the understanding of the ways in which science knowledge is constructed and how scientists go about their work over the past twenty-five years. Although in this endeavour, STS has arguably had a disproportionate influence on the study of science in society in this period.

Described as a cross-disciplinary field, and at other times as a distinct academic discipline in its own right, the history of STS is marked by a legacy of eclectic but empirically based studies of science in society. While many of these studies adopt the methods of social anthropology (described in detail in Chap. 3), there is generally a marked lack of commitment to any identifiable social theoretical position or disciplinary consistency. This is because STS research is driven by a set of problem-solving priorities stemming from 'a commitment to contest or transcend the given epistemological and/or ontological assumptions of specific historical disciplines' (Barry and Born 2013: 12). This degree of autonomy from the theoretical and philosophical perspectives of the traditional academic disciplines constituting social science has led onto the development of specialised STS undergraduate programmes, journals, and other forms of knowledge production. So that today, many prominent STS scholars see their field as a distinctive academic discipline on the basis of a common methodological approach and a distinctive knowledge base that has been built-up over more than a generation of research (Jasanoff 2016: 235). The normal expectation would be that when different disciplines come together in one field of research that there would be an accompanying range of discernable epistemological difference, but this is not the case in STS studies. This distinct lack of theoretical dispute and controversy has over time been seen as both a source of unifying strength for the field and a weakness that leads to an academic sterility.

STS research has two distinctive and characteristic methodological features. One is its implicit social constructivist reading of science and technology, often described as a 'weak' version of social constructivism in contradistinction to the 'strong' version found within SSK. This weaker form of constructivist analysis acknowledges the reality of naturally occurring phenomena alongside recognition of the importance of the social context of knowledge production. As the feminist philosopher Karen Barad has argued, 'the fact that scientific knowledge is constructed does not imply that science doesn't work' (2007: 40). The second characteristic of STS studies is their 'methodological incommensurability', the assumption that there can be no shared, objective standards for appraising scientific knowledge. STS studies therefore, generally make no judgments about the truth claims of the science work they are studying and hold the view that there are 'no external or neutral standards that univocally determine the comparative evaluation of competing theories' (Sankey 2009: 196).

The distinctive STS approach to studying the socio-cultural determinants of science work and of technological artefacts began to evolve in the late 1970s and included social scientists from North American and Western European academic institutions. What connected these studies was a shared concern to create an analytic distance from the idealised version of scientific method and practice (which it shared with SSK research in this early period), while at the same time acknowledging the materiality of science (in contradistinction to SSK). The STS approach was one that recognised the existence of a social network of scientists acting to mediate between the (natural) object of scientific research and the observational work of that scientific research undertaken by the social researchers themselves. Later still, this approach would incorporate the concerns of ANT (see Theory Box 3.1 in Chap. 3) and its attentiveness to 'the role of non-human objects in the social work of making science' (Jasanoff 2013: 103).

Sheila Jasanoff, who is cited above, is the Harvard University Professor of Science and Technology Studies and a pioneer in the field of STS. She has described the primary concerns of STS in a recent interview conducted in the *Scientific American*:

STS brings together two broad currents of research. One looks at science and technology as social institutions. How do they work and what makes them special? That, in turn, opens up many more focused questions: how do scientists and technologists discover facts and apply them; how do they decide what counts as good work; what is creativity; how do technical disputes end; how do new ideas replace old ones; and how do new scientific fields come into being? The second stream of research looks outward at the relations between science, technology and society. STS tries to understand the relationships between practices within the sciences and the interaction of discovery and invention with other aspects of society. (Horgan 2019)

Jasanoff's first 'stream' of STS research would include research concerned with exploring the role of 'representation' in scientific practice. The latter conceived as the attempt to capture, render, and otherwise make visible aspects of the world. The natural sciences are seen as having developed their own esoteric language forms and methodological logic in order to frame the natural world. One example of this type of study would be Berg's (1996) now classic research that examined the compilation of an individual patient medical record. Berg asserted that this was as much a social process as a set of cognitive processes linked to the expertise of an individual medical practitioner: 'a moulding process in which the patient and his situation are reconstructed to render them manageable within existing agency routines'. The clinician is seen to transform a patient's narrative of their illness into an entity that they as health professionals are familiar with from their training and therefore capable of managing; an activity that can be seen as unfolding 'in the doing' (Berg 1996: 502). In terms of the second 'stream' identified by Jasanoff, one recent example would be the work of Fitzgerald and Callard (2015) promoting the idea of 'entanglement'. Here researchers who study science work are encouraged not to merely stand outside (critically) looking in, but seek opportunities to work together with biomedical scientists to understand the ways in which these scientific representations are intertwined within practical experiments to produce meaningful knowledge about the 'biosocial complexities of human life' (Fitzgerald and Callard 2015: 20).

While STS studies have been extraordinarily influential in shaping an understanding of the knowledge production practices of science, there are several notable limitations associated with this approach. STS studies can be overly focused on localised and cross-sectional exchanges between science actors (both human and material); this can lead onto a neglect of the broader context in which social and economic structures serve to frame science practices over the long term. This limitation is acknowledged by Sheila Jasanoff when she states: '(W)e have to enlarge our horizons to take in the laboratories of society, where the stakes are never about knowledge alone, where values and cultural practices matter, and where power reigns through far ruder means than the accumulation of textual allies and citations' (2013: 5). A second limitation is associated with the social constructivist homogeneity of STS research. Despite its claims to the contrary, STS research often does not really 'get' interdisciplinarity in an epistemically relevant way. That is, it is rare to find a willingness to be self-critical and engage with alternative social science approaches when assessing the 'work' of science and technology. A field of research cannot be described as interdisciplinary purely on the basis of the assorted disciplinary backgrounds of its academics. It must necessarily seek to engage with and 'incorporate theories, concepts, methodologies and philosophies from diverse professional fields—a diversity of ideas reflected in the heterogeneous mind-sets of its students and professors' (Marante 2020). A final limitation is that STS research often lacks a unity of purpose, 'a clear sense of how its empirical work is, indeed, an application or, still better, a test of its theories' (Fuller 2005: 80). This lack of theory-testing is manifested in the epistemic relativism embraced by STS, in which all knowledge claims about the world are seen to be equally valid.

Scoping the Field of SSST Analytical Research

The wide scope of SSST research incorporates mainstream realist, constructivist, critical realist, and feminist philosophical perspectives; quantitative as well as qualitative research methodologies; and micro-level and large-scale comparative studies. It includes research produced by economists, medical sociologists, science historians, health economists, policy analysts, health psychologists, bioethicists, and legal analysts, as well as philosophers of science. Each of the disciplinary approaches, whether as stand-alone or in tandem with other disciplines in ITD research, has their own distinct methodological approaches to studying the knowledge production practices of the sciences and the social impact of science innovation. In order to illustrate how these differences might manifest themselves, a scenario is utilised to illustrate the range of variability and of overlap that can be found in SSST research. The scenario involves the development and marketing of a new breakthrough 'wonder' drug for treating heart disease:

1. *Health Economics*: This is a sub-field of economics as applied to health care. It is primarily concerned with how a society allocates finite resources among healthcare providers. Drawing upon economic theory, three basic questions are addressed: Which health services should be provided? How are these services and goods produced and who delivers them? And finally, who receives these goods and services and how is this allocation determined? In our example, a health economist might address the relative efficiency and effectiveness linked to the costs of manufacturing and marketing this drug. A comparative analysis with other forms of therapeutic intervention for population health improvement could be made, such as the promotion of a healthy diet and regular exercise.
2. *Medical Sociology*: This sub-field of sociology studies the physical, mental, and social components of health and illness. Key topics of research include the doctor-patient relationship; the structure and socioeconomics of health care; and cultural beliefs as they impact on the experience of disease and well-being. In terms of our example, a medical sociologist might choose to focus on individual compliance with the prescribing of this 'wonder' drug for their condition. There may, for example, have been some negative reporting of side-effects of the drug in the media; this may raise the question of where patients are situated on a trust/scepticism continuum in relation to clinical expertise.
3. *Organisational Sociology*: This sub-field of sociology examines the characteristic organising principles constituting the form and structure of particular

organisations. In terms of contextualising wider sets of social processes and also in terms of the formal and informal decision-making processes unique to the culture of these organisations. In relation to our example, the focus of research could be upon the difference in epistemic cultures co-existing in a research institute, as between a group of bioscientists and clinicians engaged in the 'bench-to-beside' development of this drug.

4. *History of Science, Technology, and Medicine*: This sub-field of history focuses on key questions concerning how scientific knowledge and the practices it has entailed have shaped and been shaped by a confluence of social, cultural, and political factors in historical societies. This understanding of the emergence of science is drawn upon to challenge, critique, or support the analysis of the present. In terms of our example, historians may choose to assess the emergence of this new therapeutic intervention in the context of the experience of failure of previous therapies hailed as 'magic bullets'.
5. *Medical Anthropology*: This sub-field of anthropology draws upon social, cultural, and linguistic difference to conceptualise the ways in which communities understand the meanings of health, illness, and well-being. This would include the experience and distribution of illness, the prevention and treatment of sickness, healing processes, the social relations of therapy management, and the cultural relevance and utilisation of health care services. In terms of our example, a medical anthropologist might seek to explore how patients conceptualise the science underpinning this pharmaceutical in the context of their shared understanding of living with heart disease. This might also involve a discussion of the construction of dependency of patients by health care professionals in the everyday management of their condition ('medicalisation').
6. *Health Psychology*: A sub-field of psychology that focuses on the behavioural factors that potentially contribute to ill-health and how psychological interventions might help change attitudes in order to prevent or effectively treat disease. In the terms of our example, a health psychologist may focus on the extent to which an individual's relative fatalism or pro-activism makes it more likely or not they will adhere to the drug regime. Psychologists may also be involved in developing behavioural change techniques to overcome perceived barriers to adherence.
7. *Bioethics*: This sub-field of ethics is concerned with the identification, study, resolution, or mitigation of conflicts among competing values or goals in the context of innovative developments in biomedicine. In terms of this particular example, a bioethicist might choose to focus on the social justice issues surrounding the decision to ration the use of this new drug because of the high cost to the health care system and how the decisions are made to include or exclude particular social groups or individuals.
8. *Public Policy Studies*: This interdisciplinary field of study examines decision-making, strategic planning processes, and interventions that are undertaken and enacted by governments in order to achieve specific (i.e., health care or science) goals within a given society. In the context of this example, a policy studies analyst might focus on the decision-making processes involved in determining that this new drug meets a recognised population health need. This process may involve the participation of 'arms-length' technological assessment body (such

as the National Institute for Health and Clinical Excellence [NICE] in the UK) in an attempt to de-politicise the funding decision-making process.

9. *Philosophy of Science*: This sub-field of philosophy is concerned with all assumptions, foundations, methods, and implications associated with the discoveries of science, their use, and merit. This involves engaging with questions of ontology (the nature of being) and epistemology (the study of knowledge and how it is achieved) when assessing the 'truth' claims of science. In the context of the example, this might involve a philosopher examining how diseases are conceptualised. That is, classifications of heart disease are constructed on the basis of clinical and epidemiological population data; these knowledge constructions may be assessed against the view that heart failure is simply the outcome of wear and tear in older age, a normal state of being in the world. If it is the latter, then questions of the utility of public investment in the development of costly treatments balanced against normative states of being are then raised.
10. *Politics of Health*: This sub-field of political science examines how questions of the power, politics, and ideology underpin health and social policy. In our example, the research focus maybe with the relative power of Big Pharma within a given society to define and address the health needs of a population outside of any system of public accountability or control.

The Structure of the Book

Given that the field of the biomedical sciences is extensive to say the least, the decision has been made to focus primarily (but not exclusively) on two of the more significant areas of research and innovation as they have impacted on society. These are the fields of genomics and neuroscience. Supporting the four chapters that assess developments within these two fields are discussions of the contribution of the philosophy of science, the gendering of biomedical science, and two chapters that engage with the governance of biomedical science research and practice.

Following this introduction to the interdisciplinary field of SSST, Chap. 2 provides an introduction to the philosophy of science. The justification for the inclusion of what some may regard as a set of esoteric concerns is that scientists hold all sorts of implicit assumptions about the natural world when they engage in the process of knowledge development. An awareness of the possibilities and limits for the formation of knowledge in a particular field (known as an epistemological question), and a concern with the nature of the being and reality of a phenomena under investigation (known as an ontological question), can help bring about the transformation of a research question in new and exciting directions. But a failure to engage in philosophical questioning of research assumptions can lead to repetition and errors. This chapter provides an outline of the philosophical assumptions underpinning the development of what we now call the 'scientific method' and includes an assessment of alternative approaches.

Chapter 3 is concerned with the research work practices of scientists. It begins by assessing Woolgar and Latour's seminal study that posed the question of how are scientific facts made in the lab? This is followed by a historico-sociological account of cell tissue culturing, as a case study of how research technologies can become 'a solution looking for a problem to solve'. The focus then turns to the question of what constitutes a scientific 'community' or 'culture'. The analysis draws on a number of case studies to describe the tensions and differences found within and between the fields of biomedical science. The chapter concludes with an examination of translational medicine and the attempts made to achieve the 'bench-to-bedside' ideal in the development of new therapeutics.

Chapter 4 begins by outlining the historical development of the cognitive neurosciences in the journey from an esoteric laboratory-based field of research to shaping the practice of psychiatry and onto direct interventions in the wider social and cultural spheres. The impact of neuro-imaging technology in revolutionising the ability of scientists to create visual representations of the working of the human brain is then examined. The chapter concludes by examining autism spectrum disorder as a case study of the relative efficacy of neuropsychiatric interventions.

Chapter 5 takes as its starting point the recent emergence of a wide array of 'neuro-disciplines' that claim to identify the neural basis of a wide variety of social and economic behaviours and processes of human development. A realist analysis of the process of 'neuro-enculturation' follows, assessing the ways in which neuroscience research is translated and utilised for commercial and political ends. Four examples of this process are examined: neurolaw, neuroeconomics, early child development, and cognitive enhancement.

Chapter 6 examines developments within the research field of human genomics. It explores the promissory research visions for radical new forms of genomic-based therapeutic interventions that followed the successful completion of the whole sequencing of the human genome in 2003, and the roles played by Big Pharma, biotechnology companies, and governments in this process. Then follows a prospective analysis of pharmacogenomics as the basis for the construction of the so-called 'personalised' system of medicine.

Chapter 7 focuses attention on the emergent biomedical research field of environmental epigenetics. It explores those 'classic' epigenetic studies that have sought to link maternal care, stress, and early development to durable long-term behavioural and disease outcomes. It then assesses the evidence for both inter- and trans-generational social effects of exposure to environmental genomic modifiers and explores the reasons why this science is often cited as a biological explanation of cycles of poverty and dysfunctional social behaviour. Despite the post-genomic repudiation of 'race' as a biological entity, it continues to be utilised as a variable in epigenetics research. This research will be critically assessed with reference to both bioethics and the methodological use of proxy measures. The chapter concludes with an assessment of the prospects for interdisciplinary health research involving epigenetic and social science, and why the definition of what constitutes an 'environment' is so crucial to its potential success.

Chapter 8 examines the processes implicated in the 'gendering' of biomedical science. The first theme assesses the neuroscience basis for the essentialising of gender that can be found in notions of the 'female brain'. It then moves onto an assessment of several examples of 'gendering' inscribed in some implicit assumptions to be found in research science. The second theme of the chapter concerns the question of why gender segregation continues to characterise careers in biomedical science.

Chapter 9 is the first of two chapters exploring the governance of biomedical science research and the constituents of 'science policy'. This chapter begins by delineating the parameters of governance and regulation; it then moves onto an assessment of the public understanding of risk associated with biomedical science innovation. It poses and addresses questions about public trust in biomedical science, and concludes with a discussion of the social and political responses to bio-disasters and the role of government in maintaining public confidence in biomedical science.

Chapter 10 draws on three case studies to critically assess the political and ethical considerations that have underpinned the construction of a regulatory framework governing the conduct of biomedical science research in the UK. Following this, there is an assessment of the emergent role of biobanks as repositories of human biological material and health data. This discussion focuses on the efficacy of bioethical principles such as informed consent and the challenges posed by the commercial exploitation of biobank data for information security and individual privacy. It concludes with an examination of the science of bioinformatics and the influential role it now plays in the processing and analysis of genomic 'big data' in society.

Conclusion: The Constituents of Critical Analysis

Generally speaking, the role of a critical social analysis is to question and challenge engrained habits of perception, understanding, and thought, and in doing so, be engaged, committed, and ultimately emancipatory in drawing attention to the possibilities for change. This is the recognition that events in the social world are never outside or completely independent from our own lives as human beings. In the context of a critical analysis of biomedical science in society, there should be a willingness to engage with any assumption that what counts as a 'natural process' or 'bioreality', is something that sits outside of the domains of the social. For it is the context of our social lives that we experience health and illness: '(B)iology and culture are mutually constraining and co-constitutive, such that they are each conditions of the others determination and development' (Slaby and Choudhury 2012: 34).

A critical analysis should also focus on unpacking what can be termed the 'black boxes' of research practice. When, for example, a particular biological process is first identified, utilising the established methods of 'logical positivism' (see Chap. 2), it may be assumed by bioscientists that this process is a regularly occurring phenomenon. A matter of fact that is settled, so that future research can be directed to improving the understanding of the inputs and outputs associated with this now newly identified biological process. However, it may be the case that the internal complexity or 'black box' element of this process are never fully interrogated. A critical analysis should always seek to be able to expand the horizons of the known (and to paraphrase ex-USA Secretary of Defence, Donald Rumsfeld) to move towards an understanding of the 'known unknowns' and even raise the possibility of knowing the 'unknown unknowns'!

Identifying the known unknowns associated with the social impact of biomedical science innovation is the primary goal of the field of SSST.

Bibliography

Allmendinger, J. (2015) *Quests for Interdisciplinarity: A Challenge for the ERA and HORIZON 2020*—EUR 27370 EN. Brussels. European Commission.

Barad, K. (2007). *Meeting the Universe Halfway: Quantum Physics and the Entanglement of Matter and Meaning*. Durham, NC: Duke University Press.

Barry, A., & Born, G. (2013). Interdisciplinarity. In A. Barry & G. Born (Eds.), *Interdisciplinarity: Reconfigurations of the Social and Natural Sciences* (pp. 2–56). London: Routledge.

Berg, M. (1996). The Practices of Reading and Writing: The Constitutive Role of the Patient Record in Medical Work. *The Sociology of Health and Illness, 18*(4), 499–524.

Berger and Luckmann. (1967). *The Social Construction of Reality. A Treatise in the Sociology of Knowledge*. London: Allen Lane; The Penguin Press.

Bhaskar, R., Danermark, B., & Price, L. (2018). *Interdisciplinarity and Wellbeing: A Critical Realist General Theory of Interdisciplinarity*. Abingdon: Routledge.

Bloor, D. (1991). *Knowledge and Social Imagery* (2nd ed.). Chicago. University of Chicago Press (Original Version 1976: London. Routledge and Kegan Paul).

Burggren, W., Chapman, K., Keller, B., Monticino, M., & Torday, J. (2017). In R. Frodeman, J. Klein, & R. Pacheco (Eds.), *The Oxford Handbook of Interdisciplinarity* (2nd ed., pp. 101–113). Oxford: Oxford University Press.

European Union. (2014). *Horizon 2020 Programme (3.1.) Societal Challenges: Health, Demographic Change and Wellbeing*. Brussels: European Commission.

Fitzgerald, D., & Callard, F. (2015). Social Science and Neuroscience Beyond Interdisciplinarity: Experimental Entanglements. *Theory, Culture & Society, 32*(1), 3–32.

Fuller, S. (2005). Is STS Truly revolutionary or merely Revolting? *Science & Technology Studie. 18*(1), 75–83.

Horgan, J. (2019, August 5). We Should All Be Science Critics. *Scientific American*. Retrieved from https://blogs.scientificamerican.com/cross-check/we-should-all-be-science-critics/.

Jassanoff, S. (2013). Fields and Fallows: A Political History of STS. In A. Barry & G. Born (Eds.), *Interdisciplinarity: Reconfigurations of the Social and Natural Sciences* (pp. 99–118). London: Routledge.

Jasanoff, S. (2016). The Floating Ampersand: STS Past and STS to Come. *Engaging Science, Technology, and Society, 2*, 227–237.

Kohler, R. (1982). *From Medical Chemistry to Biochemistry; The Making of a Biomedical Discipline*. Cambridge: Cambridge University Press.

Latour, B. (1988). The Politics of Explanation: An Alternative. In S. Woolgar (Ed.), *Knowledge and Reflexivity: New Frontiers in the Sociology of Knowledge* (pp. 155–176). London: Sage.

Mäki, U. (2016). Philosophy of Interdisciplinarity. What? Why? How? *European Journal of the Philosophy of Science, 6*, 327–342.

Marante, D. (2020). Science and Technology Studies and Its Interdisciplinarity Problem. *Areomagazine.com*, 23 July 2020.

Naughton, J. (2012). Thomas Kuhn: The Man Who Changed the Way the World Looked at Science. *Guardian*, 19 August 2012.

Porter, R. (2003). *Blood and Guts: A Short History of Medicine*. London: Penguin Books.

Sankey, H. (2009). Scientific Realism and the Semantic Incommensurability Thesis. *Studies in the History and Philosophy of Science, 40*(2), 196–202.

Slaby, J., & Choudhury, S. (2012). Proposal for a Critical Neuroscience. In S. Choudhury & J. Slaby (Eds.), *Critical Neuroscience: A Handbook of Social and Cultural Contexts of Neuroscience* (pp. 29–51). Chichester: Wiley Blackwell.

Van Noorden, R. (2015). Interdisciplinary Research by the Numbers. *Nature, 525*, 306–307.

An Introduction to the Philosophy of Science

2

Abstract

This chapter provides an outline introduction to the philosophy of science. The justification for the inclusion of what some may regard as the esoteric concerns of philosophy is that when engaged in interdisciplinary work, an appreciation of epistemological difference (concerned with the possibilities and limits for the formation of knowledge in a field) and ontology difference (concerned with the nature of being and reality) can help bring about the transformation of a research question. This chapter provides an introduction to the philosophical assumptions of realism underpinning natural science and offers an introduction to two critical perspectives of that approach, social constructionism and critical realism. Scientists hold all sorts of implicit assumptions when they engage in the process of constructing knowledge of the natural world, such assumptions necessitate engagement and interrogation, and this is a key task for the philosophy of science.

Interdisciplinarity and Philosophy

Interdisciplinary working is generally embarked upon in order to address some intractable research problems or little understood phenomenon ('known unknowns') that cannot be effectively addressed through single disciplinary research approaches. However, difficulties can be encountered when attempting to 'integrate' the knowledge assumptions of distinct disciplines. For example, sociologists, psychologists, and biologists all utilise the concept of 'health' in their research, but each theoretically contextualises the concept in quite different ways. To achieve a constructive 'inter' between two or more disciplines in ITD research requires of researchers that they pose difficult questions about the implicit philosophical assumptions of each perspective, specifically in relation to the research question that is being addressed. This involves a self-reflexivity concerning the possibilities and the limits of the

I. Crinson, *The Biomedical Sciences in Society*,
https://doi.org/10.1007/978-981-15-9523-3_2

knowledge and theory base (questions of epistemology) of each discipline. And secondly, it requires that the assumptions of each disciplinary group concerning the nature of the phenomenon being investigated and the contextual reality in which it manifests itself (questions of ontology) are brought to the surface and challenged.

An appreciation of the existence of such philosophical differences can help unpick seemingly intractable differences between disciplinary approaches that can occur in ITD work. This is a process that has been described as grasping the 'ontological imagination' (Barry and Born 2013: 19). Thorén and Persson (2013: 347) similarly point to the importance of what they term 'problem-feeding'. This is where one discipline takes on the research issues of another, and in the process of re-imagining the problem through a different epistemological lens, a potential resolution may be found. So, for example, an ITD research study exploring biomarkers for a particular health condition could involve social psychologists developing measures of psychological 'well-being' that could help construct a more nuanced conceptualisation of the impact of disease that may account for previous 'unknowns', without in anyway compromising a biomedical focus on the biochemistry of homeostasis, energy processing, or cell-cycle regulation.

In terms of making a contribution to the maximising of the effectiveness of programmes of ITD research and analysis, the philosophy of science is ideally placed as a mechanism for bridge-building, providing the intellectual tools to enable disciplinary coordination and the practice of science through the application of 'higher level' concepts. This involves the notion of 'commensurability', the understanding that science has a common language of assessment and measurement. Although it should also be recognised that a philosophical process of reflexivity can just as equally throw-up the opposite view, that of 'incommensurability'. That is, in some cases there may appear to be no shared, objective standards for establishing a scientific understanding of the research phenomenon. This is where the hard work of interdisciplinary working begins.

The Role of Philosophy in Scientific Understanding

Historically, scientific methods and theories have always been shaped by philosophical ideas whether explicitly or not. Yet this role for philosophy can sometimes be denied by modern science. The physicist and Nobel laureate Steven Weinburg has stated that, '(T)he insights of the philosophers I studied seemed murky and inconsequential compared with the dazzling successes of physics and mathematics. From time to time since then I have tried to read current work on the philosophy of science … but only rarely did it seem to me to have anything to do with the work of science as I knew it' (1992: 92). Yet Weinburg also goes on to acknowledge that '(P)hysicists do of course carry around with them a working philosophy. For most of us, it is a rough-and-ready realism, a belief in the objective reality of the ingredients of our scientific theories' (1992: 54).

Scientists generally do have a poor record in articulating the assumptions that inform their approach to studying and researching natural phenomena. Such assumptions necessitate engagement and interrogation, and this task falls to the philosophy of science. The irony of Weinburg's downplaying the value of philosophy for scientists is that in doing so, he is making a philosophical claim about how a 'realist' science should be done. Weinburg however is not alone. Many scientists still hold to the view, perhaps reflecting the singular focus inculcated in their education and training, that only natural causes can explain natural phenomena. And, that these causative processes are always essentially linear, consistent, and constant and can be empirically demonstrated. Yet, the reality of science work is that it is not simply about the accumulation of empirical data: '(I)t is about the questions we ask, the methods we employ to answer those questions, the conceptual frameworks within which we fit the facts' (Malik 2019).

But not all scientists deny the relevance of a philosophical understanding in helping focus the study of the natural world; the most eminent of these being Albert Einstein, the Nobel Prize winning physicist. In 1944, Einstein received a letter from Robert Thornton, a young African-American philosopher of science who had just taken up a teaching post at the University of Puerto Rico. He had written to Einstein with the purpose of soliciting a few supportive words on behalf of his efforts to introduce 'as much of the philosophy of science as possible' into the modern physics course that he was to teach the following spring. Einstein replied in full to Thornton as follows:

> *I fully agree with you about the significance and educational value of methodology as well as history and philosophy of science. So many people today—and even professional scientists—seem to me like somebody who has seen thousands of trees but has never seen a forest. A knowledge of the historic and philosophical background gives that kind of independence from prejudices of his generation from which most scientists are suffering. This independence created by philosophical insight is—in my opinion—the mark of distinction between a mere artisan or specialist and a real seeker after truth.* (Einstein 1944; cited in SES—Stanford Encyclopedia of Philosophy n.d.)

So what role does philosophy play in 'freeing' scientists of their prejudices? The eminent seventeenth-century English philosopher, John Locke (who was also a practicing physician and lifelong scientist), famously described the role of the philosopher in his 'An Essay Concerning Human Understanding' in the following terms: '(I)t is ambition enough to be employed as an under-labourer in clearing the ground a little, and removing some of the rubbish which lies in the way to knowledge' (Locke 1689/1975: 9). Although this notion of the 'underlabourer' appears to bring some clarity to what can be challenging issues for those engaging with philosophy for the first time, in practice this metaphor is just far too reductionist. The role of philosophy is a more proactive one than the rather limited notion of simply removing obstacles from the path to acquiring knowledge. As Peter Winch has cogently argued, the 'motive force' of philosophy is as an autonomous form of enquiry that is not dependent on the natural sciences to provide it with problems to 'solve': '(W)hereas the scientist investigates the nature, causes and effects of *particular* real things and processes, the philosopher is concerned with the nature of reality as such and in general' (Winch 1990: 8—emphasis in original).

There is a frequent misunderstanding that the role of philosophy is to construct or refute scientific theories through a priori reasoning alone. That is, to arrive at knowledge of the cause and effect of some natural phenomena purely through the application of generalised philosophical principles, without resort to empirical evidence (the assumption articulated in the quotation from Weinburg, above). The philosophy of science is not in direct competition with the natural sciences as some alternative pathway to the understanding of the world. Rather it adopts the positive role in contesting the assumptions held by scientists and in drawing out their presuppositions about the realities of the world as they engage in the practical activity of research. Philosophy therefore draws attention to the question of 'what is it to understand something, to grasp the sense of something?' (Winch 1990: 18).

It is on this basis that the philosophy of science explicitly interrogates the components of the 'scientific method' that is drawn upon in order to achieve a semblance of intelligibility about the realities of the natural world. The chapter now moves forward in outlining a critique of methodology in science.

Scientific Realism: From Empiricism to Logical Positivism, and onto the Hypothetico-Deductive Method

The idealised view of science is of a highly trained group of professionals progressing knowledge through direct engagement with the natural world through the application of a systematic investigatory approach. This view of science derives originally from the influence of the 'empiricist' philosophers of the mid to late eighteenth century, such as David Hume and John Locke (introduced above). For Hume, the process of inference of causation in the natural world is associated with the observation and identification of 'constant conjunctions'. A constant conjunction is when looking at two events, A and B, we can say that A causes B because the two always occur together. That is, whenever we find A we also find B and so have the certainty that this conjunction will continue to occur. The key philosophical assumption of what subsequent to Hume became termed 'empirical realism' is that '(T)ruths are more dependent on the natural world than upon the people who articulate them. There is a way that the world is, and it is possible to discover and represent it reasonably accurately' (Sismondo 2010: 58).

A century or so after Hume and Locke's work, a prescriptive 'scientific method' had coalesced around what was known as the philosophy of 'positivism'. Positivists adopted the position that there could only be a single scientific methodology (or 'methodological monism'), one that embodied the circular co-dependence of theory and the close observation and measurement of phenomena. This position largely held sway in the practice of science until the end of the nineteenth century. However, the self-proclaimed neutral objectivity of positivist 'scientificity', the view that scientific methods always bring a precision and certainty to knowledge, increasingly began to be questioned. This was in part due to the influence of social and political scientists such as Emile Durkheim in France and Max Weber in Germany who, in the late nineteenth century, were able to demonstrate that such scientific objectivity was in reality an illusion.

In response to this critique, a new revitalised positivist movement emerged in the early decades of the twentieth century. Now known as 'logical' or 'empirical' positivism, this philosophy re-conceived scientific method as constituted through the manipulation of the natural world and achieved through (verifiable) methods such as the experiment. Logical positivism saw the role of the scientist as gathering all possible empirical data and then exhausting all 'reasonable' considerations of what would verify their findings. Scientific knowledge was then to be generated through a process of 'Inductive inference', which drew on a rational logic to move from individual data points to hypothesised and generalised theoretical statements about the world. Scientific progress was to be achieved through the gradual improving of the correctness and range of empirical observation. Over time, the controlled experiment became the archetypal method for verifying causal inference. This method seeks to control for all variables (or at least those which can be identified) that potentially affect the process or event being studied in order to test a particular hypothesis. Within the biomedical sciences, the controlled experiment is often carried out in the form of the randomised control trial (RCT), notably in the testing of the safety and efficacy of new therapeutic drugs or clinical interventions of other kinds. The conduct of an RCT to investigate the efficacy of a new pharmaceutical drug typically involves the recruitment of a statistically representative participant sample (X) of the population, who are given either the drug to be tested or a placebo (a key aspect of the 'control' element of the experiment) over a specified timeframe. If it is found that no trial participant experiences any detectable (or at least within the timeframe of the trail) adverse side-effects, then it is reasonable to infer or extrapolate from the data that this is a 'safe' and effective drug that can be made available to the population as a whole. Inference is not certainty, but on the basis that an RCT has followed the precepts of the scientific method, it is deemed 'reasonable' to approve the safety of this drug for use in the population as a whole (Lewens 2015: 19).

While the experimental method remains preeminent within the biomedical sciences, most scientists would hesitate to draw a straight line of verification (as per logical positivism) from the 'observable' to the 'theoretical'. To do so would be naïve, given the general understanding that biases, uncertainty and limits to knowledge, will always leave open the question of the conduct of experiments, the appropriateness of the variables tested, and the inferences to be drawn. Today, there is a broad consensus that empirical data extracted from the 'natural' environment is always subject to some process of *mediation*. Hence, for a hypothesis to have any credence it must also be inherently disprovable; experimental data alone cannot constitute sufficient verification. In order to disprove a theory a scientist must *first* construct a hypotheses and then test it against experience, the current state of theoretical understanding in a particular field, as well as by observation *and* experiment; a process known as 'deductive inference'.

It was Karl Popper's (1963) work that first mounted a significant challenge to logical positivism's principles of verification and inductive inference (but not to the possibilities of realist science) by asserting that there can be no such thing as a 'pure' scientific fact derived from observations alone. 'Observation statements' were not to be trusted because they were theory-laden, reflecting a range of subjective factors as much as they were statements about what was objectively real. For Popper, theorising through inductive inference alone was essentially a process of 'imaginative creation'. He asserted that science as a 'formal activity' can only be constituted by the search for evidence to falsify a theory's prediction. This 'falsification' principle enabled Popper to place a line or 'criterion of demarcation' between genuine science and those activities he described as 'pseudo-sciences'. The latter were characterised by an inability to make firm predictions while at the same time seemingly able to explain any event/phenomena. These approaches were seen as insulating themselves from any critical examination of their methods.

For Popper, science must always proceed by a process of 'conjecture and refutation'; this is known as the hypothetico-deductive method. The scientist formulates a general claim about a natural world phenomenon and then sets about gathering evidence in an attempt to refute or falsify those claims. To demonstrate that a theory is false means a reliance upon and confidence in those observations used to refute said theory. But if observations are themselves theory-laden conjectures, then no confidence can be placed in them to irrefutably falsify a theory. Ultimately Popper did not reject but rather revised the verification principle, in establishing a new methodological standard. This new standard was a scientific method that drew on deductive inference rather than the inductive inference of classic positivism. Popper recognised that the rejection of inductive reasoning meant never being able to conclude that scientific generalisations are true, but, on the other hand, the application of deductive reasoning meant that scientists could at least conclude that some of their theories were false.

For Popper, what scientists can do at best is 'to show that one set of statements, general ones about how things work, are in general tension with another set of statements, specific ones about particular events' (Lewens 2015: 31). But how do scientists actually go about the process of gathering evidence in the attempt to falsify their own findings? In his discussion of the implicit assumptions held by many scientists today, Gezelter points out that:

> *If you ask a scientist what makes a good experiment, you'll get very specific answers about reproducibility and controls and methods of teasing out causal relationships between variables and observables. If human observations are involved, you may get detailed descriptions of blind and double-blind experimental designs. In contrast, if you ask the very same scientists what makes a theory or explanation scientific, you'll often get a vague statement about falsifiability. Scientists are usually very good at designing experiments to test theories. We invent theoretical entities and explanations all the time, but very rarely are they stated in ways that are falsifiable. It is also quite rare for anything in science to be stated in the form of a deductive argument. Experiments often aren't done to falsify theories, but to provide the weight of repeated and varied observations in support of those same theories. Sometimes we'll even use the words verify or confirm when talking about the results of an experiment. What's going on? Is falsifiability the standard? Or something else?* (Gezelter 2009)

Few if any contemporary scientist would dispute Popper's principles of deduction and falsification, yet in their purest form they would exist in a state of tension with many of the practical concerns and requirements of everyday science practice. This tension arises for the following reasons: Firstly, the existence of meaningful yet abstract scientific theories that are not systematically related to observations and so cannot easily falsified, but this does not necessarily render them irrelevant or indeed make them examples of 'pseudo-science'. Secondly, the necessity of producing promissory research visions in order to secure governmental and commercial funding often means that scientists are placed in a position where the expectation is that they should to be able to make definitive future predictions. The principle of falsification mitigates this approach. Thirdly, when theories do make incorrect predictions, the normal approach (inductive inference or 'reasonableness') in science is not to tear it up and start again, but to find explanations as to why the observations in question do not fit the theory.

Finally, it is impossible to test or falsify a hypothesis in isolation. One experimental result alone cannot tell us whether to accept or reject a hypothesis. Scientific hypotheses being dependent on a number of supporting theoretical assumptions, so even if a particular experiment appears to falsify a prediction, the experimenter can never be certain which particular set of hypothetical assumptions are now to be rejected in order to readjust this wider web of understanding. Therefore, scientists need to exercise good scientific judgement in order to decide whether to reject a hypothesis on the basis of an experimental result alone, which could be accounted for by faulty equipment, faulty calculations, or a flaw in the supporting theory (Lewens 2015: 115). This final falsification principle is commonly termed the Duhem-Quine thesis.

Thomas Kuhn: 'Paradigmatic Shifts' and 'Scientific Revolutions'

In his book, '*The Structure of Scientific Revolutions*' (*SSR*) first published in 1962, Thomas Kuhn chose to examine the history and philosophy of science from the perspective of what scientists actually *did*, rather than engage with an idealised version of the formal scientific method. In everyday life there is often a tendency to see the past through the lens of the present, and Kuhn's critique was based on the assumption that the history of science often made the same teleological error. This tendency was particularly strong in the 1960s, when the natural sciences appeared to be able to define and potentially resolve all real-world problems. It becomes a taken-for-granted assumption held by members of the public, politicians, and many scientists themselves that all scientific knowledge represented the culmination over time of a rational and progressive accumulation of theory and evidence. This conveniently ignored the discontinuous phases of research, false paths, disputes, and blind alleys that marked the actual history of science. Kuhn's historical study sought to demonstrate that in practice, scientific disciplinary boundaries have been neither entirely fixed nor fluid, but what he termed 'relational'. Relational here referring to the challenges faced by scientists when they can no longer agree amongst themselves what the key research problems are, the methods for solving them, and which core theories were able to contextualise these problems.

According to Kuhn, developments in scientific understanding are cyclical. For long periods of time, scientists in a particular field of research may share the recognition of past achievements, the essential correctness of certain core theories, what the key research problems in the field are, and the best methods for solving these problems. Kuhn termed these periods of shared understanding 'normal science'. That is, when a broad consensus is held amongst scientists about the key categories and frameworks used to understand the phenomena under investigation in any one scientific field. This framework for 'puzzle-solving' as Kuhn described it was termed a 'paradigm'. A paradigm 'acts as a guide to addressing a new problem on the basis that it is similar in type to a different problem that we already know how to solve' (Lewens 2015: 80). Failure to solve a particular problem would then be seen as reflecting the quality of the research rather than the paradigm itself. A paradigm can serve to 'insulate the community (of scientists) from those socially important problems that are not reducible to the puzzle form, because they cannot be stated in terms of the conceptual and instrumental tools the paradigm supplies' (Kuhn 1970: 37).

However, at some point anomalies in research findings begin to accumulate and take on the character of real problems not puzzles per se; this is what Kuhn termed the period of 'crisis'. Such crises arose because scientific paradigms can at best only be ever partial representations of reality. The response within a scientific discipline to such a crisis is what Kuhn describes as being a 'non-cumulative developmental episode' or 'paradigm shift'. Rejecting the old exemplars, new theories begin to emerge which can account for the previous research anomalies. If scientific paradigms shape scientific observations, then as the previously dominant paradigm is replaced, so scientist's beliefs about the phenomenon they are observing must also necessarily change. Research conducted under the now rejected paradigm then becomes 'semantically incommensurable' with the new position, so that the meaning and terms of reference found in the previous paradigm cannot now be mapped onto the terms used in the new paradigm (Baghramian 2013: 273).

Kuhn was later forced to row-back on some of his stronger claims about scientific incommensurability in the light of further studies of apparent revolutionary moments in the history of science. These studies demonstrated that while the meanings of scientific terms certainly did change following a paradigm shift, they did not systematically change to the point where the older paradigm could not be understood or compared with the new. However, more modest claims about semantic incommensurability could be substantiated. There is now more evidence available to demonstrate that scientists frequently fail to effectively communicate with one another on what should be a common point of science, even on essentially the same subject matter. Kuhn (1970) also later acknowledged, in the second edition of his *SSR*, that he utilised the concept of a 'paradigm' too broadly and not always in mutually reinforcing ways. His working definition of a scientific paradigm was what members of a particular scientific community were seen to have in common. He expanded this definition in the second edition of *SSR* in order to embrace; 'the entire cluster of problems, methods, theoretical principles, metaphysical assumptions, concepts, and evaluative standards that are present to some degree or other in the concrete, definitive scientific achievement' (Orman 2016: 49). This acknowledged lack of specificity in the first edition opened up Kuhn's concept of paradigm shift to criticism, re-interpretation, and misinterpretation. It is therefore more productive to see the notion of paradigm shift as a heuristic device rather than as a bounded theoretical concept. That is, as a 'rule of thumb', an analytical tool to shed light on a set of complex processes rather than being a precise analysis of epistemic difference within science.

In summary, *SSR* profoundly changed the direction of thinking within the philosophy of science in two major ways. Firstly, the assertion that changes in scientific theory are not historically progressive, nor solely driven by data (and the accompanying process of inference), but derive from radical and discontinuous new scientific visions of the world. Secondly, the thesis that scientific communities are organised around the practice of paradigm-building which in turn serve to shape scientist's interpretations of natural world phenomena in a particular field of research. It is on this basis that Kuhn's approach is usually described as 'constructivist'. So it is to the post-Kuhnian philosophy of science, and in particular, the position of social constructivism and its denial of the possibilities of achieving a realist science that we now turn.

Anti-realism: The Social Construction of Knowledge in Science

Anti-realist philosophy is concerned with switching the 'how' questions of realist science around and begin rather than end with the process of knowledge construction of the natural world. The key philosophical assumption is that abstract hypotheses and scientific laws cannot exist within an intellectual vacuum that is cut off from the presuppositions, accumulated epistemic experiences, and practical requirements of doing science work. The very existence of a biomedical science, for example, presupposes a history of establishing knowledge-cognition practices enacted through the training and socialisation of an epistemic (shared knowledge base) culture or community of scientists (discussed in detail in Chap. 3).

Anti-realism is especially critical of classic accounts of the process of scientific discovery that idealises 'eureka moments' in the search for 'truth concerning the unobservable' (van Frassen 1980: 5—cited in Sismondo 2010: 63). An anti-realist philosophy of science conceives research as a constructive process, in the practical 'geometrical sense' of the attempt to make sense of the fixed points of data emergent from experimental observations. For Knorr Cetina, the existence of heterogeneous, differentiated, and discrete 'cultures of knowing' in science poses a challenge to the realist view of a homogeneous application of the hypothetico-deductive method across all fields of science research:

> *(T)he practical success of science depends more upon the scientist's ability to analyse a situation as a whole, to think on several different levels at once, to recognize clues, and to piece together disparate bits of information than upon the laws themselves. As with any game, winning depends less upon the rules than with what is done within the space created by those rules.* (Knorr Cetina 1981: 3)

In research practice, scientists are seen to make decisions about the frameworks of understanding they will draw upon *prior* to making their observations. So that while scientific theories are in principle inductively inferred by reference to the data arising out of empirical observations, in practice they are not always implied by that data. To put it yet another way, while representations of nature are connected to nature they do not necessarily correspond to it in any strong sense (Sismondo 2010: 64). Anti-realists point to the necessity for scientists to engage in a process of construction and contingency when engaged in theorising natural phenomenon; a redefining of scientific objectivity in relativistic terms. On this point, Christopher Norris has argued that:

> *(F)or talk of truth the anti-realist would substitute talk of empirical adequacy, epistemic warrant, or 'truth' (what presently counts as such) relative to some conceptual scheme, framework, discourse, paradigm, research programme, or whatever. For talk of objective or mind-independent reality they would likewise substitute one or other of a range of favoured substitute conceptions whereby objectivity is redefined in terms of what is taken to merit that title according to our optimal or current-best perceptual, cognitive, epistemic or scheme-relative means of ascertainment.* (Norris 2014: 8)

A central critique of the anti-realist philosophy of science is that it: 'reacts to regularity theories of causation by throwing out causation instead of the regularity assumption, if it ignores the possibility that reasons or discourse can be causal, then it simultaneously rejects the means of understanding how we can be architects rather than bees' (Sayer 1997: 475). Anti-realism therefore has a tendency to a reductive relativism, that is, conceiving all science phenomena as social constructions whether this be a biological mechanism or the first draft of a scientific paper for publication. As indicated in the quotation from Chris Norris above, anti-realism has its own implicit or 'contrastive working notion' of scientific 'truth'. It draws upon this understanding when identifying the errors and false pathways down which realist science travels in its own search for truth. One particularly difficult issue for anti-realism to confront is that the realist method of science is frequently successful in developing and applying explanatory models in predicting events and processes in the natural world. This is sometimes termed the 'no miracles' position.

Finally, it should be acknowledged that the vast majority of scientists do in practice recognise a clear distinction between having knowledge of, and the 'truth' about, a particular natural phenomenon. All working scientists know through experience that science knowledge is often error-prone, historically situated, and frequently incomplete. The notion of a 'scientific truth' is always going to be 'verification-transcendent', that is, going beyond what the scientific method itself is designed to achieve (Norris 2014: 17).

So far in this chapter we have looked at the emergence of a realist philosophy of science which moved in defined historical phases from a narrow empiricism to logical positivism then onto the hypothetico-duductive principles established by Popper. In more recent times, the understanding of what constitutes the scientific method has been challenged by an anti-realist philosophy built on constructivist principles. The latter has been particularly influential within STS-informed studies of science work (discussed in Chap. 1). Further below, a rather different philosophy of science known as critical realism will be outlined. However, prior to that, in the form of a concise summary, five key analytical points of comparison between these philosophies of science are set out in the form of a matrix in Table 2.1. These five comparative dimensions are (a) Ontology, (b) Epistemology, (c) Methodology, (d) Explanation, and (e) Theory.

Table 2.1 Philosophies of science in five key dimensions (I.C adapted from Fleetwood 2013)

	Realism: Positivism and empiricism	Anti-Realism: Constructivism and idealism	Critical Realism: Stratification and emergence
Ontology	• Reality as observable events. • Closed systems not open.	• Realities as relativistic and socially constructed. • Scientific entities cannot exist independently of their identification. • Identification derives from discourse, language, and signs.	• Reality as hierarchically stratified. • Three domains of reality: Empirical; Actual; Deep. • Emergent powers at each level of strata that cannot be reduced to that below.
Epistemology	• Knowledge derives from observable events. • Causality is event regularity. • Truth derives from hypothesis testing.	• The primacy of epistemology over ontology. • No separation of ontology (conceived as flat, not stratified) from epistemology. • 'Truth' is relativistic	• The primacy of depth ontology over epistemology. • The fallibility of knowledge. • 'Truth' about a natural phenomenon or event by empirical means alone will always be partial, situated, and provisional
Methodology	• Covering law method. • Laws are event regularities (not tendencies) = closed systems	• Deconstruction • Historical genealogy.	• Causal-explanatory. • Objective is to explain not derive causal laws.
Explanation	• Causal explanation is prediction.	• What is explained is not a scientific entity/event itself, but the ways in which it is socially constructed.	• Explanation not prediction, as latter impossible in complex real-world open systems
Theory	• Vehicle for predictions	• Sceptical of theory	• Vehicle for causal-explanatory accounts

Critical Realism: Ontological Realism and Epistemological Constructionism

As discussed in relation to the history of STS (in Chap. 1), the 'science wars' of the early 1990s involved a number of prominent natural scientists in a public 'roughing-up' of the constructivist assumptions held by SSK academics. Their view was that these constructivist accounts represented a denial of the possibilities for undertaking objective science and this had to be challenged. These scientists made little distinction between the anti-realist philosophy of science found in SSK and other non-constructivist social scientific critical assessments of the methods of normative science (Segerstråle 2000). But beyond the heat of these 'science wars', an internal opposition to strong forms of constructivism was already building within the field of SSK. These new approaches took a number of distinct epistemological forms. One pathway was that taken by what was to become Actor Network Theory (see Theory Box 3.1 in Chap. 3). Another pathway, which had its origins in a more overtly philosophical interdisciplinarity, was that of Critical Realism (CR). The distinctive CR philosophy of science combines an ontological realist understanding of the natural world with an epistemological constructionism concerning how the knowledge of that real natural world emerges. At first sight these two pillars of CR appear to constitute a logical contradiction; below we will assess whether this is in fact the case.

The first of these two pillars, 'ontological realism', reflects the CR recognition of the existence of a stratified world, a recognition that is derived from the scientific understanding of the evolution of life on this planet. The established reality of the natural world exists independently of perceptions and theories and is seen to consist of hierarchically organised layers or strata, with physical mechanisms in one stratum, chemical mechanisms in another, biological in a third, with psychological and social strata being at the top of this hierarchy. Moving upwards through these strata of reality:

> *We find that each new stratum is formed by powers and mechanisms of the underlying strata. At the same time, this new stratum represents something entirely new, unique and qualitatively different, which cannot be reduced to underlying strata. When the properties of underlying strata have been combined, qualitatively new objects have come into existence, each with its own specific structures, forces, powers and mechanisms.* (Danermark et al. 2002: 60)

It is on this basis that Roy Bhaskar, one of the leading figures in the early development of CR, argued that society is irreducible to nature and likewise individuals to their biology. That is, the new non-reducible properties and mechanisms that are added at the level of each specific strata of reality must be understood in terms of new or 'emergent powers' (Bhaskar 1989). The idea of emergence is crucial for CR, so that to see the natural and social world purely in empirical terms (what can be measured and observed) is seen to be misleading because it reduces what is (the ontological) to what we can know about it (the epistemological). Bhaskar (1978) has described this methodological error as the 'epistemic fallacy'.

Identifying the scientific processes, powers, and mechanisms that are emergent at each level of strata points to the necessity of adopting interdisciplinary approaches when contextualising causality, for example, at the biological and the social levels when assessing some aspect of humanity. The question of which mechanisms are the most significant for a particular object of scientific study can only be decided from case to case, through empirical studies, and in relation to the research problem that is being addressed. This philosophical understanding of the existence of a 'depth reality' clearly presents a challenge to those scientific positions that have traditionally rested upon single causative factor explanations of natural phenomena. So, for example, is it hereditary genetics or environmental factors that most pertain in health outcomes? Or is it evolutionary biology or social conditioning that determines or shape human behaviour? These and many other examples of foundational or essence-type causal explanations to found in the natural sciences, including biomedical science, are directly challenged by a CR understanding of stratification and emergence (Danermark et al. 2002: 62–63).

The second assumption or pillar of CR is that any scientific (or indeed lay person's) conceptualisation of the natural world consists of constructions, so that every attempt to empirically grasp this complex reality is necessarily simplified and incomplete. Developing a knowledge of reality can only be attained if we go beyond what is empirically observable. This is achieved by asking questions about and developing concepts of the mechanisms and processes corresponding to different levels of reality from which events and phenomenon are emergent. However, and this is where the constructionism necessarily arises in CR, the knowledge that is attained of that world is always going to be 'fallible and transfactual, and its usefulness varies under different conditions' (Danermark et al. 2002: 22). Scientific laws of causality are seen as transfactual, that is, 'the more or less universal preconditions for an object to be what it is' (Danermark et al. 2002: 77). But the scientific method frequently attempts to capture natural processes in isolation, in a closed system of experimentation structured by human intervention. So there can be no certainty that the powers, potentials, and liabilities of these natural processes may or may not be actualised or indeed manifest themselves in completely different ways within open systems, outside of scientific study. In real world open systems, constant conjunctions are not always forthcoming in ways predicted by scientific generalisations. Posing this epistemological question of how best to identify and capture generative processes and mechanisms in natural (and social) objects has particular relevance when validating and evaluating research findings. But this CR critique of the scientific method has nothing common with the relative constructionism of anti-realism (Danermark et al. 2002: 25).

Bhaskar (1978: 56) has set out what he calls an 'ontological map' or hierarchy of three domains of scientific reality which forms the basis of the CR philosophy of science; a slightly modified version of this original 'map' is set out in Fig. 2.1. The first rung of hierarchy is the empirical domain of direct experience. This is the characteristic domain of scientific experimental practice that seeks to produce 'data' or 'facts', through the perception and observation of the existence of 'dependent' and 'independent' variables, facilitated by the construction of closed system mediated by theoretical conceptions. As Bhaskar explains, 'an experiment is necessary

Domain	Entity	Ontology
Empirical	Experiences and Perceptions	Flat
Actual	Events and Actions	
Depth Reality	Structures, Mechanisms, powers, relations	Depth

Fig. 2.1 An ontological domain map of science realism. (Adapted from Bhaskar 1978)

precisely to the extent that the pattern of events forthcoming under experimental conditions would not be forthcoming without it' (1978: 33). So the oft-used expression, 'the empirical world', is a fundamentally misleading one. We then move onto the second domain of the 'actual', where events and actions happen, whether or not we experience or observe them. What occurs within this domain is not necessarily the same as that which is observed in closed system of experimentation. Finally, the domain of 'depth reality'. This domain produces events in the world, both natural and social, seen in terms of emergent powers and generative mechanisms pertaining to each distinct strata (Danermark et al. 2002: 20).

This ontological map represents the 'crux' of Bhaskar's critique of empirical realism, as an approach to science characterised by a 'flat ontology'. Empirical science is seen to constitute 'an ontology based on the category of experience, as expressed in the concept of the *empirical* world and mediated by ideas of the *actuality* of the causal laws and the ubiquity of constant conjunctions, three domains of reality are collapsed into one' (Bhaskar 1997: 57). This understanding is what distinguishes critical realism from other forms of realism in the philosophy of science.

This chapter has focused on the reasons why an understanding and familiarity with the conceptual frameworks of philosophy are so important in the undertaking of research science. Questions of ontology and epistemology do really matter in any critical evaluation of the outcomes of science work.

Chapter Summary: Key Points

- *Achieving an 'inter' between two or more disciplinary approaches requires questions to be posed at not just the epistemological level, but also at the level of ontology.*
- *The philosophy of science can provide the intellectual tools to enable interdisciplinary coordination through the application of 'higher level' concepts.*
- *Scientists generally have a poor record in articulating the implicit epistemological assumptions that inform their approach to studying natural phenomena.*

- *The 'motive force' of philosophy is as an autonomous form of enquiry that is not dependent on the natural sciences to provide it with problems to 'solve'.*
- *Philosophy engages with science when it draws attention to the question of what is it to understand something, to grasp the sense of something?*
- *'Logical positivism' conceives science as constituted through the manipulation of the natural world achieved through (verifiable) methods such as the experiment.*
- *Today, there is a broad consensus that empirical data extracted from the 'natural' environment is always subject to some process of mediation.*
- *Karl Popper—'Observation statements' about the natural world are not to be trusted as they are theory-laden, reflecting subjective factors as much what is objectively real.*
- *Thomas Kuhn—Science work is organised around building paradigm-relative social practices that then serve to shape interpretations of natural world phenomena.*
- *Anti-realism—Science as a constructive process, in the practical 'geometrical sense' of making sense of fixed points of data from experimental observations.*
- *Critical realism—Combines ontological realism with an epistemological constructionism, points to emergence and generative powers existing at the level of depth reality.*

Bibliography

Baghramian, M. (2013). Relativism about Science. In S. Psillos & M. Curd (Eds.), *The Routledge Companion to the Philosophy of Science* (2nd ed., pp. 268–179). London: Routledge.

Barry, A., & Born, G. (2013). Interdisciplinarity. In A. Barry & G. Born (Eds.), *Interdisciplinarity: Reconfigurations of the Social and Natural Sciences* (pp. 2–56). London: Routledge.

Bhaskar, R. (1978). *A Realist Theory of Science* (1st ed.). Hassocks: Harvester Press.

Bhaskar, R. (1989). *The Possibility of Naturalism: A Philosophical Critique of the Human Sciences*. Hassocks: Harvester Press.

Bhaskar, R. (1997). *A Realist Theory of Science* (2nd ed.). London: Verso Press.

Danermark, B., Ekström, M., Jakobsen, L., & Karlsson, J. (2002). *Explaining Society: Critical Realism in the Social Sciences*. London: Routledge.

Fleetwood, S. (2013). *What Is (and What Isn't) Critical Realism*. Centre for Employment Studies Research (CSER) Seminar, 20th September 2013—University of the West of England.

van Frassen, B. (1980). *The Scientific Image*. Oxford: Clarendon Press.

Gezelter, D. (2009). Being Scientific: Falsifiability, Verifiability, Empirical Tests, and Reproducibility. *The Open Science Project*. Retrieved September 2017, from http://open-science.org/.

Knorr Cetina, K. (1981). *The Manufacture of Knowledge: An essay on the Constructivist and Contextual Nature of Science*. Oxford: Pergamon Press.

Kuhn, T. (1970). *The Structure of Scientific Revolutions* (2nd ed.). Chicago: Chicago University Press.

Lewens, T. (2015). *The Meaning of Science*. London: Pelican Books.

Locke, J. (1689/1975). An Essay Concerning Human Understanding. In P. Nidditch (Ed.), Oxford. Oxford University Press.

Locke, J [edited by Nidditch,P] (1689/1975). An Essay Concerning Human Understanding. Oxford. Oxford University Press.

Malik, K. (2019). Einstein Got It Right—Philosophy and Science Do Go Hand in Hand. *The Guardian*, 24 February 2019.

Norris, C. (2014). What Strong Sociologists Can Learn from Critical Realism: Bloor on the History of Aerodynamics. *Journal of Critical Realism, 13*(1), 3–37.

Orman, R. (2016). 'Paradigm' as a Central Concept in Thomas Kuhn's Thought. *International Journal of Humanities and Social Science, 6*(10), 47–52.

Popper, K. (1963). *Conjectures and Refutations*. London: Routledge.

Sayer, A. (1997). Essentialism, Social Constructionism, and Beyond. *The Sociological Review, 45*(3), 453–487.

Segerstråle, U. (2000). Science and Science Studies: Enemies or Allies? In U. Segerstråle (Ed.), *Beyond the Science Wars* (pp. 1–34). New York: State University of New York Press.

SES—Stanford Encyclopedia of Philosophy. (n.d.). *Einstein's Philosophy of Science*. Retrieved September 2019, from https://plato.stanford.edu/entries/einstein-philscience/.

Sismondo, S. (2010). *An Introduction to Science and Technology Studies* (2nd ed.). Chichester: Wiley-Blackwell.

Thorén, H., & Persson, J. (2013). The Philosophy of Interdisciplinarity: Sustainability Science and Problem-Feeding. *Journal for General Philosophy of Science, 44*(2), 337–455.

Weinburg, S. (1992). *Dreams of a Final Theory: The Search for The Fundamental Laws of Nature*. New York: Random House.

Winch, P. (1990). *The Idea of Social Science and Its Relation to Philosophy* (2nd ed.). London: Routledge.

Laboratory Studies, Epistemic Cultures, and the Routines of Scientific Work

3

Abstract

This chapter is concerned with the process that scientists engage in the laboratory, beginning with an assessment of Woolgar and Latour's seminal study that first posed the question of how are scientific facts made? This is followed by a historico-sociological account of the science of cell tissue culture, described as 'a technology solution looking for a problem to solve'. The focus then turns to the question of what constitutes a 'scientific community'? The key characteristics of what are termed 'epistemic cultures' are described, using illustrative case studies describing tensions and difference found within and between the fields of bioscience. It concludes with an examination of translation medicine, examining the interprofessional and disciplinary tensions that emerge attempting to achieve the 'bench-to-bedside' ideal.

Introduction

Laboratories are often represented as a demarcated or bounded space, separating the worlds of science and everyday life. This is where the 'formal' work of scientists is enacted through the methods of experimental science. As scientific knowledge and practice came to be seen as a legitimate object of sociological enquiry, so social scientists became attracted to the possibilities of conducting anthropological studies of scientists at work in their 'natural habitat'. This chapter describes and assesses the contribution of 'laboratory studies' as they became known and how they shone light on the pragmatic approach to experimentation adopted by teams of scientists, frequently marked by uncertainty and informal understanding. The chapter moves onto assess what are termed the 'epistemic cultures' in more detail in a case study of the tensions existing between two fields of biology, systems and synthetic

I. Crinson, *The Biomedical Sciences in Society*,
https://doi.org/10.1007/978-981-15-9523-3_3

biology. The chapter concludes with an assessment of translational medicine, drawing on three case studies to examine why 'gaps' occur in the different phases of research associated with moving from 'bench-to-bedside'.

Anthropologists in the Lab

> *It takes an anthropologist in the laboratory to note the strangeness of what has become quickly routinized or banal to its practitioners*. (Landecker 2007: 3)

Latour and Woolgar's (1979) '*Laboratory Life*' was the first major example of an up-close study of the work of scientists in a laboratory. This was an early example of STS-orientated study (see Chap. 1 for a detailed outline) that drew on an ethnographic methodology. Ethnography is a qualitative research method that involves the researcher 'immersing' themselves in the day-to-day activities of a social group or community. Empirical data is collected, but the primary focus is to describe the culture, ecology, and belief systems of the social group under investigation. Latour and Woolgar's approach consistent with social anthropology was to treat the scientists as an 'alien tribe'. The idea being that if these scientists were viewed as 'aliens', then the researchers could not impose their own presuppositions on what they were recording and observing. What were unfamiliar laboratory practices for these social researchers would allow them to pose naïve and direct questions that the scientists as experts in their field would not normally expect to be asked. More generally, the study sought to focus on the issue of how science facts are made? And, in what ways did laboratory work give stability to scientific claims about an object of scientific analysis so that it comes to constitute accepted knowledge about that natural object?

The following lengthy but revelatory quote from the study gives a flavour of the ethnographic approach that was adopted:

> *Our anthropological observer is confronted with a strange tribe who spend the greatest part of their day coding, marking, altering, correcting, reading, and writing ... our observer has begun to make sense of the laboratory in terms of the tribe of readers and writers who spend two-thirds of their time working with large inscription devices (see Glossary). They appear to have developed considerable skills in setting up devices which can pin down elusive figures, traces, or inscriptions in their craft work, and in the art of persuasion. The latter skill enables them to convince others that what they do is important, that what they say is true, and that their proposals are worth funding. They are so skillful, indeed, that they manage to convince others not that they are being convinced but that they are simply following a consistent line of interpretation of available evidence. Others are persuaded that that they are not persuaded that no mediations intercede between what is said and the truth. They are so persuasive, in fact, that within the confines of their laboratory it is possible to forget the material dimensions of the laboratory, the bench work, and the influences of the past, and to focus only on the 'facts' that are being pointed out. Not surprisingly, our anthropologist observer experiences some dis-ease in handling such a tribe. Whereas other tribes believe in gods or complicated mythologies, the members of this tribe insist that their activity is in no way to be associated with beliefs, a culture, or a mythology. Instead, they claim to be concerned only with 'hard facts'. The observer is puzzled precisely because his informants insist that everything is straightforward. Moreover, they argue that if he was a*

scientist himself, he would understand this. Our anthropologist is sorely tempted by this argument. (Latour and Woolgar 1979: 69–70)

The site of the study was a team of research scientists engaged in the isolation and characterisation of the chemical structure of thyrotropin-releasing hormone (TRH), which has a central regulating role in metabolism, blood pressure, and other crucial functions of the body (see Glossary). The objective of this research was to attain the structure of TRH so that a synthetic compound could be produced and compared with the original, ultimately for clinical application. The genesis of this 'new object' occurred over an eight-year period, and involving two separate laboratory-based research groups. These research groups led, respectively, by Schally and Guillemin, published between them a total of forty-one papers concerned exclusively with identifying the structure of TRH. Both research groups were subsequently to be awarded the 1977 Nobel Prize in Medicine for their discoveries concerning peptide hormone production in the brain.

Latour and Woolgar's observations emphasised the drawn-out nature of the 'stabilisation' processes associated with extracting a single purified structure for TRH, out of the many other equally probable structures. This process involved repeated bioassays (see Glossary) of purified sheep and pig brain extracts, with each new experiment redefining the range of possible explanations of the structure of TRH. The final isolated chemical structure (not a simple polypeptide as initially thought) with consistent qualities then became the 'solid fact' of TRH. In this iterative process of testing, the micro-social interactions and negotiations between scientists in the laboratory were seen as playing a crucial role in the day-to-day management of a fraught and challenging research programme. A synthetic replica of TRH, 'R-Glu-His-Pro', was actually produced by the research team before knowledge of the natural TRH had been constructed from the bioassays. The use of synthetic chemistry had proven to be sufficient by itself to narrow down the possible sequences of TRH from six to one, 'without having to touch the precious micrograms of the natural extract' [*extracted with great difficulty from many metric tons of pigs and sheep hypothalami*] (Latour and Woolgar 1979: 144).

At this point in the scientific endeavour, the two research groups agreed that the synthetic compound had the same biological action as natural TRH but not that TRH had the structure 'R-Glu-His-Pro'. However, providing a satisfactory answer to the problem of evaluating the differences between the synthetic and natural materials remained. Mass spectrometry was seen as providing the definitive answer to this question and to avoid further scientific argument and conflict. One of the lab teams eventually succeeded in introducing a natural sample of the brain extract into a mass spectrometer (there had been overwhelming difficulties in achieving this technical goal until very late on in the research programme), and to obtain a spectrum that, 'no one in the field could interpret as being significantly different from that for the synthetic material. This was the first example of the structure of a natural product being determined on the basis of its similarity with a synthetic product' (Latour and Woolgar 1979: 147).

Latour and Woolgar tended to view that many of the observed practices of scientists appeared to be similar to the everyday routines to be found outside of the context of the laboratory. They concluded that there was no simple answer to the question of how science facts are made in lab work but rather emphasised the 'indexical' nature of data collection in experimental work. Scientific facts were seen to those 'objectified' results that followed a long process of negotiation among colleagues, exploring what the date they have produced following experimentation actually represented. On this basis, Latour and Woolgar made the assertion that the meaning of a research object (TRH) only becomes clear when the science can be transformed into a social object (the negotiations and interactions between scientists). By observing scientific work close-up, ethnographic studies do not assess whether a claimed scientific fact is valid or not, but rather what are the understandings of the scientists themselves, in the light of their experimental findings.

In a later re-evaluation of *Laboratory Life*, Latour (1987), whose work was by now informed by Actor Network theory (see Theory Box 3.1), moved away from idea of the research object being a social object. He now argued that scientific data was constructed through 'networks', where the scientist-experimenter is just one element in a process that brings together colleagues from a range of disciplines (biologists, chemists, physicists, etc.), and crucially, material and other technical objects such as laboratory apparatus, theories, and subjects (in the case of TRH, this would be the brain extracts of animals) to produce 'inscriptions'. The latter being the visual or representational records of this experimental 'set-up' that can then be taken away from the lab and worked upon, and combined with many other inscriptions, to finally produce a coherent scientific argument and published scientific paper. The process of moving from the pragmatic and iterative experimental methods of a team of scientists, often marked by uncertainty and informal understandings, to the writing of a scientific paper setting out the process in terms of formal scientific language has been described as a process of 'translation' and condensation. This final published scientific paper rarely if ever records the informal human scientist interactive processes, the failed lines of enquiry, and the shared discussions over paradigmatic principles.

A further conclusion that can be drawn from this anthropological research is that knowledge derived from laboratories is knowledge about things that are distinctly non-natural. A position that in part derives from the fact that the materials used within laboratories, that is, cell lines, knockout mice, and so on, are all pre-prepared. They are standardised, purified, and even enhanced before being subjected to experimental manipulation; there is often also an assumed predictability of the chemical interactions involved. For the observer from the outside world, the laboratory can be seen to be 'a site of action from which "nature" is as much as possible excluded rather than included' (Knorr Cetina 1983: 126).

In contradistinction to the positive presentation of the ethnographic approach adopted by Latour and Woolgar, a realist assessment of their position as outsiders in the laboratory is that they do not see what the scientists saw. What scientists may recognise as data of significance are often difficult to identify as distinct objects or clear readings for non-experts. Not surprisingly, scientists as experts have learned through their training and professional socialisation to read their material in a way that novices cannot. However, at the same time, the ethnographic research finding that experts often see what they believe to be relevant does open the door to the suggestion they may be missing other interesting features of their material (Sismondo 2010: 108).

Realist social studies of laboratory work unsurprisingly tend to be less focused on how scientific objects are constructed and more focused on the empirical side of lab work. Mark Erickson's (2016: 36) research examined the work of a team of molecular biologists engaged in the field of bacterial genetics. His concern was to study the differences between the experimental activities of the team and the information that was included in their write-up of the research process. As Erickson notes, the published paper describes plasmid (see Glossary) construction in just a couple of paragraphs, yet none of the complex, meticulous, and patient laboratory benchwork required to produce these findings is mentioned in the published paper (2016: 47). Equally, the experimentation that led onto the generation of an innovative bacterial gene splicing technology, involving ten separate complex steps and nine months of work for the main investigator and three other team members, was reduced to an explanation of just 106 words. As Erickson concludes; '(L)aboratory work is a bit like an iceberg: the visible portion is what can be seen in the publication or conference presentation, but beneath that tip there is a massive amount of preparatory work, failed experiments, grant writing, meetings, ordering lab supplies, writing draft papers, emailing colleagues in different parts of the this thought community, and so on' (Erickson 2016: 56).

▶ Theory Box 3.1 Actor Network Theory There are internal disagreements as to whether ANT is a theory per se, or a method of inquiry, but this is essentially a semantic distinction given that theory and methodology are necessarily entwined. What is clear is that despite the epistemological differences with SSK (see Chap. 1), ANT shares with the latter a commitment to an anti-realist philosophy of science (see Chap. 2).

ANT views knowledge as 'embodied' not only in the shared understandings of social actors, but in a wide variety of material forms; 'test tubes, reagents, organisms, skilled hands, scanning electron microscopes, radiation monitors, other scientists, articles, computer terminals, and all the rest' (Law 1992: 2). But where does this 'knowledge' come from? John Law provides the following answer: '(Knowledge) is the end product of a lot of hard work in which heterogeneous bits and pieces … from the social, the technical, the conceptual and the textual are fitted together, and so converted (or "translated") into a set of equally heterogeneous scientific products … (and) what is true for science is also said to be true for other institutions … the family, the organisation, computing systems, the economy and technologies—all of social life—may be similarly pictured' (Law 1992: 2).

ANT seeks to map out the relations existing between these 'heterogeneous bits' or 'ensembles' (the term 'entanglement' is also widely used in ANT research to describe the same construct) that includes human agents, technology and other material objects, and conceptual ideas. Whether these 'bits' are human or non-human does not matter, all are seen to be 'actors within a network of connectivity'. Here the term 'actor' should not be read as (human) 'agency' or intentionality, as is usual in sociology, but refers to the effects of these ensembles or the impact of their presence in a given social context. Latour developed this position with his assertion that the 'social' cannot be construed as material or as a distinct domain but rather 'designates what is *already* assembled together' (2005: 1) He goes to argue that any attempt to distinguish between the material and the social makes little sense since they are 'inherently inseparable': '(T)here is no social that is not also material and no material that is not social' (Latour 2005: 1). It is for this reason that the 'social' prefix before 'construction' is rejected in ANT.

ANT-informed research is typically focused on these network connections that are made and remade between human and non-human entities, in a range of science contexts. John Law sets out this position straightforwardly as follows: '(ANT) is a toolkit for telling interesting stories about how relations assemble' (Law 2002: 203).

In the words of Bruno Latour, the notion of 'nature' like that of 'society' conflates two different functions: '(O)n the one hand, the *multiplicity* of beings making up the world; on the other the *unity* of those assembled in one single undisputable whole. Appealing to realism is never enough, since it means throwing together in one package multiple matters of concern as well as unified matters of fact … what the two collectors, nature and society, have in common (is that) they are both premature attempts to collect in two opposite assemblies the *one common world*' (Latour 2005: 254—emphasis in original).

Transforming Life in the Laboratory

Hannah Landecker's *Culturing Life* (2007) is a sociological-historical account of the development of in vitro tissue culturing in the laboratory over the course of the twentieth century. She begins her book by noting that:

> *The life form of the cultured cell is a manifestly technological one: It is bounded by the vessels of laboratory science, fed by the substances in the medium in which it is bathed, and manipulated internally and externally in countless ways from its genetic constitution to its morphological shape. Its existence bears little resemblance to the body plan or the life span of the organism from which its ancestors were derived …. (But) because of this familiarity*

we have forgotten how to ask the basic question, how can life once firmly seated in the interior of the bodies of animals and plants be located in the laboratory? (Landecker 2007: 3–30)

The first successful attempt at culturing cell tissue occurred in 1907, with Ross Harrison's nerve tissue experiments in the USA. Harrison's techniques were subsequently adopted and elaborated by Alex Carell in 1910. This breakthrough in the in vitro technique of tissue culturing represented a prominent example of the process of modernisation that was occurring within the biomedical sciences at the beginning of the twentieth century. The new technical ability to move beyond the limitations of in vivo experimental practice to promote the culture of cell tissue in the lab enabled 'plasticity'; 'the pushing and pulling of biological things to live in different shapes and spaces and times, to be practically realized through the manipulation not just of the cell tissue itself but the medium in which in lives' (Landecker 2007: 11).

Having established that the technique of in vitro culturing of cell tissues was a practical achievement, Harrison's research moved into a new phase involving a collaborative partnership with Carell. Their work in the 1920s was focused on culturing embryonic chicken heart tissue, with the goal of achieving 'immortality' for cells. Carell had consciously chosen heart tissue to culture to 'illustrate the possibility of endlessly renewed life, with its manifest liveliness—the rather uncanny ability to pulse stop pulsing, and start over again in the space of a few day' (Landecker 2007: 76). In this pursuit of 'biological infinitude', Carell is seen as driven by the idea of transforming the fantasy of immortality found in novels and poems, into material form within his laboratory. The technique of cell tissue culturing is also a good illustration of a process that is not uncommon in the history of bioscience research. That is, a new technology is developed with no obvious immediate application and so becomes 'a solution looking for a problem to solve'. It was not to be for another forty years, before this 'solution' was fully to be realised, in the culturing of human cell lines on a mass scale in the laboratory for use in testing vaccines. In 1951, the first human cell line was established in the USA and was named 'HeLa' after a young women, Henrietta Lacks, who had become the unwitting donor of a sample of her cancerous cervical tissue taken for a regular biopsy. The sample was used without her express knowledge or consent to culture a strain of human cells for laboratory use; in perpetuity (Landecker 2007: 139). HeLa cells subsequently enabled a successful national testing process for a vaccine for polio to be carried out and enabled tissue culturing to become a standardised practice within biomedical laboratories for many decades to come.

From the very beginning, tissue culturing came to stand for more than just the material thing itself (the cell tissue) reproduced for the first time in the laboratory. Tissue culturing not only represented the successful development of in vitro experimentation, but also introduced the practice of 'visualisation' for the first time. Carell successfully pioneered the use of time-lapse cinematography in the 1920s precisely in order to capture the movement of nerve endings in the dimension of time. This cinematography meant that the 'wonders' of this new culturing technique could be demonstrated to a much wider audience than colleagues in a laboratory. Together, these developments fundamentally shifted the perceptions of biomedical scientists, 'from what had been inside … the physiological notion of interiority and invisibility, to the very visible and autonomous existence of tissue cells in the laboratory setting' (Landecker 2007: 61). It also represented a new and profound realisation for bioscientists that from now on the scientific experiment 'was no longer bounded temporarily by a finite survival period … (and) an organism was no longer the only location for the reproduction of cells to make tissues' (Landecker 2007: 72). This autonomy from the body and seemingly immortal existence of tissue cells was subsequently to pose challenging social and ethical questions that remain to this day.

The Epistemic Cultures of Science

In Chap. 2, we looked at the work of Thomas Kuhn (1970) and his understanding of the role played by scientific paradigms in linking scientists within a field of research. Kuhn's work was influenced, although he did not explicitly acknowledge it as such, by Ludwig Fleck's (1935/1979) conception of 'scientific thought communities', published forty years earlier. Indeed, Fleck's contribution to the conceptualisation of scientific communities was not widely appreciated until 'rediscovered' in the late 1970s. Fleck was a microbiologist by training but became interested in why sociologists (of the 1930s) chose *not* to see scientific knowledge as an object of legitimate social analysis, seemingly standing outside of social and cultural processes. His own view was that the work of scientists 'did not exist in, or emerge from a vacuum' (Erickson 2016: 149). While Kuhn's work on scientific paradigms is rooted in the philosophy of science and in history, Fleck's is a sociological account (predating social constructionist theories) of the ways in which communities of scientists bring the social into the production of knowledge.

Fleck recognised that whether engaged in everyday activities or in scientific research, the processes of cognition are enhanced through shared activity. What he termed a 'thought community' was essentially a group of individuals who shared ideas, concepts, and more formalised theories. The 'thought style' of science communities is collectively held and shared and constitutes the basis upon which facts are identified and validated. Being a member of a scientific thought community meant not only sharing a common scientific knowledge base, but also adopting a 'style of thinking' that relied on seeing the wider social world in similar ways (Erickson 2016: 96).

Fleck's work also predates that of Michael Polanyi (1958), whose philosophical understanding of the role of 'tacit knowledge' in science practice remains influential to this day. In undertaking his analysis of the complex decision-making processes characteristic of science work, Polanyi concluded that process involved not only the high level of expertise embedded in the professional training of scientists, but also a sharing of something unique to that community. He identified this unique characteristic as the unexpressed and perhaps inexpressible elements which together constitute what is termed 'tacit knowledge' (Jacobs 2006: 170). Polanyi defined tacit knowledge as belonging to the scientist as a 'thinking knower', but this was an 'unarticulated knowledge' never expressed in formal terms in research papers and books. The notion of 'tacit' implies that the steps taken from one part of a research problem to addressing the whole could not easily be explained. The scientist is seen at first to be orientated solely on the research problem at hand, but then they are seen to shift 'attentiveness away from individual entities toward a complete entity in which they are combined in a manner that we cannot define' (Polanyi 1985: 30). This process is seen to reflect the 'active forming of experience during the process of acquiring knowledge' (Polanyi 1985: 15).

Drawing on the sociology of scientific knowledge, Harry Collins (2010) in his book, *Tacit and Explicit Knowledge*, sought to tease apart Polanyi's umbrella term and identified three distinct meanings of scientific tacit knowledge as follows:

(a) Relational tacit knowledge: knowledge that is in principle, explicable, even if for some reason or another it is not explicated. The relevant information is simply obscured or withheld by the scientist. Collins quotes a scientist who he had interviewed for his research to illustrate this point: 'Let's say I've always told the truth, nothing but the truth, but not the whole truth'.
(b) Somatic tacit knowledge: This is embodied knowledge in the sense of learning to ride a bike, but also in terms of the physical skills ('feel') required in the use of laboratory equipment to clone an antibody, for example. Such knowledge can potentially be made explicit, but it is not the distinctive root of scientific knowledge per se.
(c) Collective tacit knowledge: This is knowledge as embedded in the material context and intellectual arrangements found in a particular laboratory, that is, 'learning on the job'. For Collins, the acquisition of knowledge is essentially tacit in science work when it is tied to social interactions in the laboratory.

Polyani's recognition of the tacit elements of scientific knowledge and Collin's later iteration of the concept are both acknowledgements of its robustness and grounding in shared human expertise; this is not knowledge that can be digitalised. Collective tacit knowledge is a necessary acquired expertise that enables scientists to 'break out of the experimenter's regress (see Glossary). Scientists with tacit knowledge can transmit their technical expertise, unadulterated, through interactional intermediaries, but they cannot reduce such knowledge to an algorithm' (Doing 2011: 304). The work of Fleck, Kuhn, and Polanyi serves to challenge the simplistic mainstream view of scientists as 'thinking knowers', unique possessors of finely calibrated scientific minds. The concept of tacit knowledge is a useful device for pointing to the existence of multiple forms of knowledge that are irreducible to one another in the shared practice of a community of scientists.

The work of Karen Knorr Cetina informed by an ANT perspective, adopts a rather different tack. Her concern is 'not in the construction of knowledge but in the construction of the machineries of knowledge construction' (Knorr Cetina 1999: 3).

On this basis, what are described as 'epistemic' or knowledge cultures of science work are seen to act; 'like *ensembles* of sense and memory organs and manipulation routines onto which intelligence has been *ascribed*' (Knorr Cetina 1999: 99—emphasis in original). These 'epistemic cultures' are seen as encompassing 'networks of practices, arrangements, and mechanisms bound together by necessity, affinity and historical coincidence, that in a given area of professional expertise, make up how we know what we know' (Knorr Cetina 2005: 69).

Epistemic Disputes in Interdisciplinary Bioscience: The Case of Systems Biology

In this section, we will explore the tensions and disputes that can arise when new epistemic communities emerge to challenge established boundaries within science work. The discussion draws on sociological research assessing the significance of epistemic difference from the viewpoint of bioscientists themselves, as they reflect on their everyday research practice. This section takes account not only of the social interactional aspects of science work, but also organisational factors and so includes but moves beyond a social constructionist analysis.

The discussion brings together the findings of two research papers, both involving interviews with scientists drawn from the field of systems biology and the related field of synthetic biology. These fields of research represent relatively recent developments in bioscience and which on the surface appear to represent a radical divergence from the mainstream molecular approach of bioscience. Systems biology is an interdisciplinary approach that brings together biologists, physicists, mathematicians, engineers, and computer scientists with the aim of making biology as quantitative and predictive as physics. The idea of 'calculating life' is the ultimate aspiration of many scientists in this field. The field of synthetic biology seeks to take the aspirations of systems biology still further, by introducing engineering principles with the objective of constructing living systems. The process of computer modelling biological systems involves what are termed 'high-throughput' "-omics" techniques (see Glossary). These technologies are sophisticated computational tools, able to generate large-scale data sets on the DNA, RNA, and protein levels. The data sets are integrated to enhance information extraction in order to model biological processes as interconnected and regulated networks in silico (D'Argenio 2018: 1). Note: The role of bioinformatics in the analysis of 'Big Data' now generated by genome sequencing and other large-scale molecular data-gathering techniques is discussed in detail in the context of biobanking in Chap. 10.

The first paper by Jane Calvert and Joan Fujimura (2011) is based on interviews with over fifty scientists working in the systems biology field in the UK, Japan, and the USA. Three features of the work of systems biologists that are seen to mark a significant divergence from more traditional bioscience emerge from this qualitative research. The three 'divergences' are seen as the interdisciplinarity built into the working environment of systems biology, a holist approach to doing biology, and greater intellectual rigour.

In terms of the first of divergences, as we have seen in the social analysis of laboratory work above, there are two distinct elements in play in the work of scientists, the technical-epistemic and the social, and the work of systems biologists is no exception. The epistemic element is the application of the 'high-throughput' computing techniques described above, while the social elements relate to the challenges of interdisciplinary team working. The interconnectedness of these social and epistemic elements in the work of systems biologists can be seen literally in the glass-encased open-plan laboratories that are increasingly physically incorporated into the architecture of modern biomedical research centres: 'These new buildings have interdisciplinarity purposely built into their design, and incorporate social spaces and "streets" to encourage serendipitous interactions between "wet" experimental and "dry" computational researchers' (Calvert and Fujimura 2011: 156). Working in this new type of open-plan research environment with wet labs immediately adjacent to computing facilities can be challenging for those scientists who have been trained in more traditional forms of bioscience research practice, described as 'comfort zones' or 'silos' by the scientists in the interviews. Nevertheless, these innovations in both the organisation and the physical environment in which the work of systems biology is carried out 'may be the most important way (it) is different from the life sciences that preceded it' (Calvert and Fujimura 2011: 157). One example of this new form of 'interdisciplinary design' would be the Francis Crick Institute in Central London. This opened in 2016 and now employs 1500 scientists and support staff working collaboratively across a range of disciplines, making it 'the biggest biomedical research facility under a single roof in

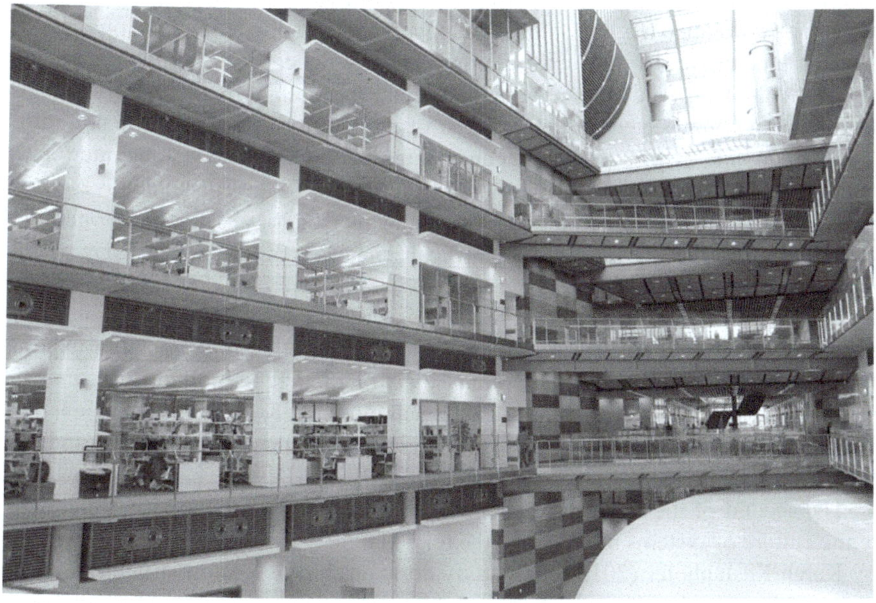

Fig. 3.1 Open-plan lab spaces inside the Francis Crick Institute—© Francis Crick Institute

Europe'. Figure 3.1 shows these open-plan research spaces in which systems biologists engage in their interdisciplinary working practices.

The second epistemic divergence identified in Calvert and Fujimura's study concerns the veracity of the claim made by the systems biologists in the interviews to represent a more 'holistic' way of doing biology than the 'reductionism' of traditional molecular biology. The systems biologists typically claimed that molecular biology only attends to the functioning of the microbiological aspects of the whole human organism such as DNA or proteins. In contrast, they claim to focus on how these molecular 'parts' become organised into 'systems'. Indeed one of the scientists claimed that systems biology could be defined as 'the study of emergent properties' (Calvert and Fujimura 2011: 158). The discourse of anti-reductionism also emerged in the interviews, possibly reflecting the need to further distinguish the field from molecular biology for funding and other purposes. Yet, the accusation of reductionism levelled at molecular biology can only go so far. In practice, systems biologists begin with the same molecular-level data and then attempt to map from the bottom-up, the components of whole systems. As such, there is just a different form of reductionism at work in systems biology, one that replaces molecular reductionism with that of mathematical reductionism (Calvert and Fujimura 2011: 159).

The third divergence identified in the study is the claim of the interviewees to be more quantitatively 'rigorous' than the 'intuition or naïve understanding' seen as a characteristic of molecular science. This belief is based on the application of a very different set of epistemic elements more usually to be found within mathematics and the physical sciences, focusing on the discovery and application of laws and systems-level principles using computer modelling (Kitano 2004: 826—cited in Calvert and Fujimura 2011: 159). The strength of this modelling approach applied to biology is claimed to give systems biology the potentiality to improve prediction. Not the prediction of biological processes already understood through the use of conventional lab-based research methods, but the ability to predict something unknown and unexpected. In the grandest of terms, this is the goal of making life itself 'calculable'. However, Calvert and Fujimura also found that some interviewees (they termed 'dissenters') offered a different view of the epistemic divergence of systems biology from the practices of molecular biology. They questioned the assumption that the standards of the physical sciences were the standards by which they should now measure their achievements in systems biology. In fact, the majority of the systems biologists who were biologists by training rather than as computer scientists recognised the key role played by 'wet' biology in conducting experiments at the laboratory bench rather than solely on modelling biological systems in silico. These trained biologists were also much more likely to express the view that systems biology was a progression of biological understanding rather than indicative of a paradigm shift (Calvert and Fujimura 2011: 161).

The second of the research papers explored in this section exploring the epistemic culture of systems biology and the related field of synthetic biology is written by Karen Kastenhofer (2013). This study drew on thirty-six semi-structured interviews with researchers from both these fields of bioscience, supported by additional observations and documentary analysis. The objective was to 'delineate differences and similarities, incompatibilities and blurred boundaries' between the approaches of systems and synthetic biology often framed as within the literature as being 'two sides of the same coin'. Both groups of scientists were seen to exhibit varying degrees of reluctance to categorise themselves as systems or synthetic biologists in the interviews: '(S)ome scientist's prefer to state they "do" systems or synthetic biology, while conceiving of themselves as biochemists, molecular biologists or computer scientists' (Kastenhofer 2013: 133). It was found that both fields were engaged in the process of epistemic community building through the establishment of specialised conferences, textbooks, taught curricula, and other outward-facing constructions.

Kastenhofer identified the existence of what she termed 'grand visions' for each of the fields. For the synthetic biologists, this was to bring engineering into biology, while for the systems biologists, there was found to be a vision of developing a 'tool box' for the study and comprehension of natural systems. Yet both groups of scientists were tentative about whether computer modelling in practice was able to build not just reliable in silico models, but actually to replicate complete living systems and not just because of the limitations of the computing technology then available. This is because all living organisms interact with an environment that is subject to change over time and so lack a finite number of elements that can be modelled. In other words, the reality of biological systems is that their complexity, flexibility, and globalisation do not lend themselves easily to analysis by binary computing systems (Kastenhofer 2013: 137).

Both of these realist-orientated research papers found the epistemic cultures of systems biology to have a material-organisational as well as ideational base. While the epistemic differences within this field of bioscience are certainly tangible, as divergent disciplinary traditions come together (voluntary or otherwise) in interdisciplinary practice, these differences may turn out to be more flexible and complimentary than has been suggested in constructivist accounts of science communities. The reality of the interdisciplinary research-built environment and the requirements of the research funders for 'deliverables' can be seen to overcome any apparent incommensurability between the distinct traditions (biology, maths, physics, engineering, and computing), methods, technologies, and skill-sets that together constitute the field of systems biology. Yet as this adoption and adaption process within interdisciplinary research continues, 'new questions emerge for systems biologists about what constitutes biological understanding, what a biological question is, and even what we should recognise as a biological object' (Calvert and Fujimura 2011: 11).

Models of Disease in Laboratory Work

The experimental models of disease that are drawn upon in laboratory work usually fall into one of three broad categories, which are informed by a fourth type—the molecular biology of the genome. These are in vitro cell culture (discussed above);

traditional animal models of disease, for example, in relation to hypertension, arthritis, cancer, or multiple sclerosis; and mouse models involving various types of gene knockouts, knock-ins, and their variants. While the congruence between in vitro and animal models of disease and some corresponding human condition has long been a fundamental assumption of research practice, in more recent years this understanding has come under critical scrutiny.

Horrobin's (2003) work poses several important questions concerning the ability of these disease models to produce the informational outcomes required for the translation of laboratory-based findings into effective therapeutic interventions. In relation to in vitro modelling, Horrobin asks does the functioning of cells in culture bear a sufficiently strong relationship to the functioning of cells in an organ in vivo such that conclusions drawn from the former are useful in predicting behaviour of the latter? His answer is that an important distinction must be made between the anatomical and functional biochemistry of the cell as follows:

> *It is reasonably safe to say that if a particular biochemical step is present in vitro, then that particular biochemical step is also likely to be present in at least some form in vivo. We can therefore construct a network of all possible biochemical events in vivo by examining all possible biochemical events in vitro. But what the in vitro system cannot do is construct a functional and valid in vivo bio-chemistry. And that is potentially a fatal flaw. For in most human diseases it is the functional biochemistry and not the anatomical biochemistry which goes wrong. When we ask cell culture to inform us about in vivo cell function, in most cases we ask too much.* (Horrobin 2003: 152)

In relation to animal models of disease, the question that is posed is does the use of animal models of disease take us any closer to understanding human disease? Horrobin's conclusion is that with rare exceptions, the answer is likely to be negative given that animal models can only be congruent with human disease when both are fully understood in all key respects. The assertion is that these conditions have not been fulfilled for any human disease. Even in infectious disease research, 'the animal model is often very different from the supposed human disease because of differences in the immune response' (Horrobin 2003: 152). In relation to mouse models of disease, the question that is posed is will genetically modified mice lead to better understanding of human disease? Horrobin's view is that most human disease is highly unlikely to be due to a single abnormal gene and that consistent phenotypes are rarely obtained for laboratory research by modification of the same gene even in mice. This is relevant because the great majority of human diseases that affect large numbers of the population are likely to be the result of the interaction of several different genes (Horrobin 2003: 153).

Carrie Friese's (2013) anthropological research concerned with the use of animal models raises further questions about the assumptions of consistency that are central to the requirement for standardisation and reproducibility in experimental science. Friese identifies the often neglected (at least within published scientific research) but crucial role played by laboratory staff in 'caring' for experimental animals. Such 'care' is critical to accurate, reliable, and translatable findings, but its presence in experimental work, as a set of tacit knowledge and skills (see above), has long been repressed. These research observations led Friese to identifying the care of lab animals as a 'potentialising practice' for a science. Note: further to the application of animal models, the use of rodents in epigenetic research is discussed in Chap. 7.

Bench-to-Bedside: The Translational Imperative in Biomedical Research

> *The medical benefits of the current revolution in biology clearly cannot be achieved without vigorous and effective translation. Yet the triple frustrations of long timelines, steep costs, and high failure rates bedevil the translational pathway.* (F. Collins 2011)

As discussed in Chap. 1, the conception of 'biomedicine' arises from the coming together of biochemistry and clinical medicine in the early years of the twentieth century. This integration of two distinct epistemic traditions reflected the increasing dependence of clinicians on innovations in tissue testing for effective patient diagnosis, combined with the increasing opportunities that newly developed pharmaceutical medicines offered to intervene at the level of biochemical and metabolic processes in human disease. The 1960s witnessed an exponential increase in commercial and governmental funding to identify so-called magic bullets to address the increasing prevalence of cancer, cardiovascular and other degenerative diseases. Today, what is termed 'translational' research has arguably become the core activity of biomedical science.

The primary objective of translational research is to bridge the gap between the ever-expanding knowledge base of the molecular biological sciences and the requirements of clinical medicine for innovative and effective tools for disease management. Yet new therapeutics have not come on stream at the pace predicted by the advances achieved in the basic biomedical sciences, reflecting the practical difficulties involved in achieving the 'bench-to-bedside' ideal. In the USA, despite billions of dollars of research funding, less than 25% of highly promising biomedical discoveries resulted in a published randomised clinical trial, and less than 10% of that total were rolled out in the form of therapeutics in clinical practice within twenty years (Drolet and Lorenzi 2011: 2).

The concept of 'translation' loosely describes the transformation of knowledge through successive fields of research, a process that requires both laboratory-based research (benchwork and clinical trials) and non-research activities (implementation). Figure 3.2 is a representation of translational activities occurring along a linear continuum or pathway. In this diagram, these translation activities are represented

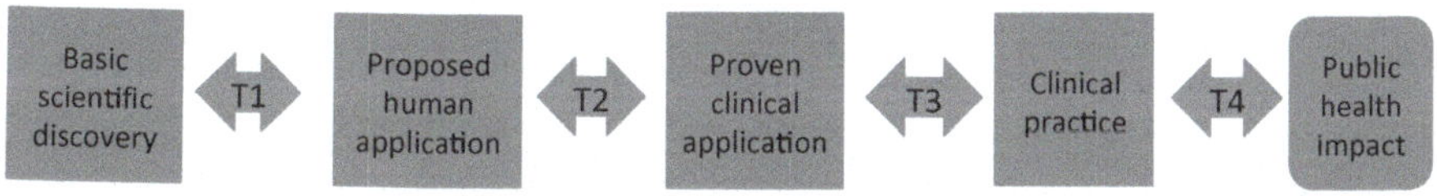

Fig. 3.2 The bench-to-bedside translational pathway

in an unproblematic one-directional flow of information from basic scientific discoveries (T1) in the laboratory through different phases of clinical trials (T2) and onto application in clinical medicine (T3). The final phase (T4) represents the implementation of diagnostic guidelines for health system take-up ultimately leading onto improvements in population health.

In practice, the difficulties faced in achieving success in translational research are far more complex than the pathway illustrated in Fig. 3.2. Translation frequently represents a dilemma for research bioscientists. They are fully aware of the simplifications and reductions that their experimental work necessarily requires but are increasingly expected to achieve a rapid applicability of their findings. Orientating basic research towards the goal of the development of therapeutic applications has over time become an imperative for biosciences research. The 'Mission & Scope' Statement of the academic journal '*Science Translational Medicine*' states that

> *Studies in humans often highlight deep gaps in our fundamental understanding of biology, but the linkages back to basic research to fill these gaps have not been as effective as they could be. Clearly, creative experimental approaches, novel technologies and new ways of conducting scientific explorations at the interface of established and emerging disciplines are now required to an unprecedented degree if real progress is to be made. Nothing short of a true reinvention of the science of translational medicine is likely to suffice to aid in this reinvention.* (*STM*—accessed Sept 2019)

Figure 3.3 identifies the 'gaps' that research activities are required in practice to bridge at each translational point (T1, T2, etc.). The 'zone of translation' is the term given to the sum total of activities that must occur before impact on public health can be achieved. At Gap T1, interpretation of a basic bioscience discovery must be made in the context of a potential clinical medicine application. At Gap T2, after a potential human application is identified, animal studies and subsequently human clinical trials are required to evaluate the safety and efficacy of the interventions. Gap T3 is only bridged when clinical practices and guidelines are implemented and adopted within health care systems, while Gap T4 reflects the potential gap between

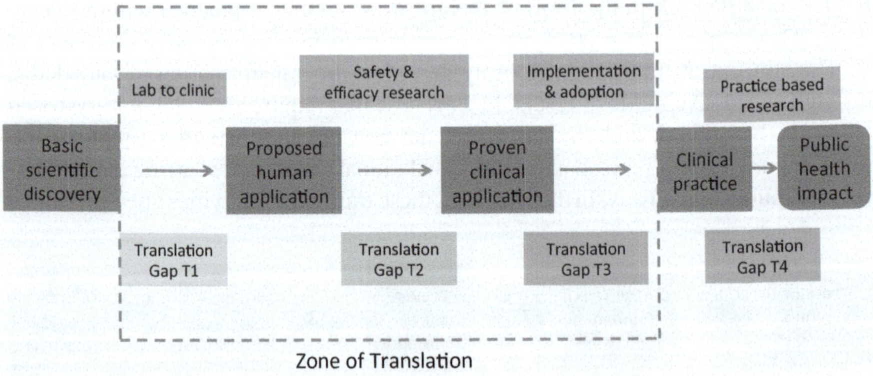

Fig. 3.3 Biomedical research translation and gaps

the new clinical applications as they are rolled out and their actual impact on population health outcomes.

The identified gaps in the phases of the translation process essentially 'represent "black boxes" in which activities of translation remain vague' (Drolet and Lorenzi 2011: 4). The broader the gap that requires bridging, the 'more complex and multifarious' translational research becomes. From this perspective, translational research is not just about the translation of one kind of knowledge (scientific discovery) into another kind of knowledge (clinical effectiveness), but is also concerned with the practical development of medical and pharmaceutical technologies, changing professional practice and ultimately improving health for patients. When translational research is conceptualised too narrowly, 'it risks losing sight of what is necessary to make knowledge or applications valuable for individual users and society' (van der Laan and Boenink 2015: 38).

Translation research can also therefore be conceptualised as a 'hybrid-practice' (Keating and Cambrosio 2003), one that brings together a range of 'social actors', including bioscientists, professionals, and organisations, including technicians, doctors, bioscientists, policy-makers, funders, and regulators, for the purpose of achieving the 'translational imperative' (Abi-Rached et al. 2010: 13). To explore the outcomes and repercussions of this interactivity in more detail, it is useful to look at the findings of three case studies of translational research in practice.

The first example is an ethnographic study conducted by Harrington and Hauskeller (2014), which drew on interviews and observations with members of a research team engaged in a Phase One Trial designed to develop stem-cell treatments for clinical implementation ('The British Cardiovascular Collaborative for Stem Cell Repair of the Heart'). What emerged from the study were the deep tensions existing between the 'clinician-scientists' and molecular scientists in the team. These tensions were seen as arising from the differing attitudes of these scientists, as distinct epistemic groupings, towards the translational process. The view of the bioscientists was that the process was essentially an adjunct to biological inquiry; they conformed to the 'translational imperative' only in order to get research funding, while the clinical scientists adopted the unsurprising position that biological research should be driven by clinical requirements. As one of the clinicians interviewed in the study states: 'all agreed that clinical researchers had first to define which problems they would attempt to treat with transplanted cells and by what route. Then the groups working on animal models would adapt their models to that clinical need' (Harrington and Hauskeller 2014: 197). The ethnographic study concluded by noting that the research collaborative group ceased meeting together in 2012, having worked together for a seven-year period. The reason for the split was that the clinical scientists had shifted their research focus to work on a different clinical trial that involved the use of established stem cells. This, the authors suggest may be interpreted as a case where the tensions between biological and medical research could not be resolved and where the translational imperative failed to generate new treatments as originally envisaged.

The second case study is Levin's (2014) ethnographic study of a translational research programme in metabolomics (the post-genomic study of the molecules and processes that make up metabolism) with an intended application in clinical surgery. This study highlights the 'non-linear and often problematic attempt to create, shape, and move data between the realms, conceptual and physical, of laboratory research and clinical practice' (Levin 2014: 93). As was noted in Chap. 2, 'data' defined as a series of techniques and practices is neither neutral nor self-evident; it always requires interpretation and translation to be scientifically meaningful. On this basis, Levin argues that the differing contexts of the laboratory and of the surgery clinic constitute not only different 'realms of practice', but also different ideas about what constitutes disease. The approach of the bioscientists in the research programme was to devise computational algorithms and sequences of code, to look for patterns within their biochemical data. Their concern was not with the biological composition of tissues per se, but rather with demonstrating statistical relationships present at the molecular level (a 'molecular signature of anatomy'). The clinicians, on the other hand, found this use of data to develop 'molecular maps' of disease particularly challenging. Their professional socialisation had led them to view that in addition to acquiring a biomedical knowledge base, clinical practice also necessarily involved elements of experience, judgement, and interpretation. Their surgical background therefore led them in a different direction from that of the bioscientists. They eschewed the digitally generated molecular maps in favour of the analogue qualities found in histopathology tissue slides to identify whether morphological markers of vascular invasion or tumour grade and stage in order were present. These different uses of data led to different interpretations of the potential to translate metabolomics technologies for use in clinical practice. As Levin concludes, translational research 'relies on the interpretative abilities of medical practitioners jut as much as data' (Levin 2014: 106).

The tensions deriving from the differing epistemic assumptions of biomedical scientists and those of clinicians engaged in translational research also emerges in a third case study. This ethnographic interview-based research conducted by Brosnan and Michael (2014) examined the activities of a neuroscience research group trialling therapeutics for Parkinson's disease (PD) patients. The site of this translational research programme was within a university attached to a hospital, with the research team located on two floors under the same roof. On one floor were the labs where 'wet' science was carried out. This involved testing the effect of a protein on the proliferation of natural stem cells taken from foetal rat brains. The second floor consisted of a carpeted waiting room and a suite of consulting rooms where the clinician researchers assessed the cognitive functioning of patients taking part in a long-term study of PD. The scientists and clinicians were effectively functioning as separate groups but formally bound by the prefix 'neuro' in their research activities. Interviews were conducted separately with the lab-based and clinically based research staff. And from these interviews emerged, perhaps not too surprisingly, two distinct epistemic versions of the 'neuro-reality' of Parkinson's disease. Below are some extracts taken from the interviews with the laboratory-based and the clinical research staff members as they appear in the study.

The interviewer asks both the laboratory-based researcher (LR5) and the clinical researcher (CR1) the same question in turn. Note the ways in which both resisted the idea of a coherent unitary neuroscience or a shared disciplinary gaze:

Interviewer: *Do you think neuroscience as a whole, raises any particular ethical issues?*

LR5: Neuroscience? What do you mean by neuroscience?

Interviewer: *Well I mean, as opposed to other areas of bioscience.*

LR5: What do you mean? What do you mean? Neurobiology, or, neurology? I mean, that's two different concepts to me. I mean, neurology is to deal with neurological conditions in patients, but neurobiology is to deal with neuro-logical symptoms in experimental models in cells or in animals or whatever. So I mean, what do you mean by neuroscience?

Interviewer: *Do you see yourself as working in neuroscience? How would you describe your work?*

CR1: I guess I am working in neuroscience. But, for me, the most important part of it is meeting the patients … so although it is neuroscience, I wouldn't really be cell based, more kind of psychology based, neuropsychology.

This is a good example of the ways in which the formal coherence of neuroscience as a field of research was questioned by both groups engaged in the translational research. This interdisciplinary unity was questioned by one of clinician-scientist leaders (GL) of the research project, who made the following comment:

GL2: And there's no time to read. Like you open the *Journal of Neuroscience*, you have cellular neuroscience, disease neurobiology, behaviour, cognitive systems biology, systems neuroscience, and you see how you skim through, and you say, 'Oh well in this section, cognitive neuroscience, I'm not going to bother to read any of this because, I don't know, it's not in my frame of thinking'.

What was clear from these and other interviews with members of both research groups presented within this study was that a common basis in neuroscience on its own was not enough to bridge the epistemic and professional cultures of the lab and the clinic. However, this did not mean that the ultimate goal of translation was denied. In fact, the translational research group as a whole was found to function effectively because of the presence of an overarching logic at work. This 'logic' was the ability of the research Group Leader (GL), a clinician-scientist (a clinician with a strong background in laboratory science), to act as the glue in the project. The GL was found in this study to have succeeded in 'adhering' the two parts of the research group together. They were able to do this through presenting a clear prospective vision for the research group as a whole:

GL1: Historically, what we've done is we've spent a decade describing aspects of disease, both Parkinson's and Huntington's disease, and we've spent a decade in the lab trying to better understand behaviour of transplants and innate repair mechanisms. And I think, for me, the future is now how can we make that into a, a more unified approach—experimental therapeutics. So, for me, the next ten years will be much more about not just describing what goes on in the disease, but trying to alter it, so actually trying to push for therapies more to the clinic, and to try and think of what we can do in the lab which will have a much clearer input into the clinic. So I think having described, we now have to explain. And once we've explained, we can then interfere.

While the Group Leader had a clear vision for the translation pathway, adopting what he described as 'experimental therapeutics', the team members were less certain in their responses to what was being 'translated'. Nevertheless, they saw the Group Leader as an embodiment of the 'neuroscience' that underpinned the research project. The role of the Group Leader was to make lab work relevant to the clinic and vice versa: 'If it is the GL who is uniquely positioned to "do" translation, there is no need for others to invest too much thought in how it proceeds or, indeed, what it practically entails' (Brosnan and Michael 2014: 694). The clinician-scientist becomes the embodiment (the 'logic') of a 'together but apart' adhesive form of organisation, translating the work of the lab into clinically efficacious interventions (Brosnan and Michael 2014: 694).

The conclusion that can be drawn from all three of these case studies of translational research in action is that for such research to have a reasonable chance of being successful, it requires some sort of unifying individual or incentive sitting above that of the epistemic cultures of the participating groups of clinicians and bioscientists.

Chapter Summary: Key Points

- *As scientific practice came to be seen as an object of sociological enquiry, so many social researchers were attracted to the possibilities of conducting research within laboratories.*
- *Ethnographic studies of science work do not assess whether a claimed scientific fact is valid or not, but rather what scientists themselves understand about their activities.*
- *The history of tissue culture is both a history of ideas and the material things in and through which conceptual change occurred (Landecker* 2007*: 26).*
- *Cell culturing is an example of technology developed with no immediate application, a solution looking for a problem to solve.*
- *Scientists with tacit knowledge can transmit their technical expertise, unadulterated, through interaction with others, but cannot reduce such knowledge to an algorithm.*

- *Epistemic or knowledge cultures encompass networks of practices and mechanisms bound together by necessity and affinity that make up 'how we know what we know'.*
- *Epistemic differences are tangible, but as fields come together in interdisciplinary practice such differences may turn out to be much more flexible and complimentary.*
- *Effective communication across disciplines in ITD can be achieved when scientists are 'sensitised to the co-existence of different epistemic values'.*
- *Horrobin (*2003*) asks does the use of animal models take us any closer to understanding human disease? With rare exceptions, the answer to this question is likely to be negative.*
- *The concept of translational research describes the transformation of knowledge through successive phases of research, known as the 'zone of translation'.*
- *The broader the gap that requires bridging, the more 'complex and multifarious' translational research becomes.*
- *Tensions in translational research practice often derive from the differing epistemic assumptions held by biomedical scientists and those of clinicians engaged in the process.*

Bibliography

Abi-Rached, J., Rose, N., & Mogoutov, A. (2010). *Mapping the Rise of the New Brain Sciences*. Working Paper BIOS no. 4. London. LSE.

Brosnan, C., & Michael, M. (2014). Enacting the 'Neuro' in Practice: Translational Research, Adhesion and the Promise of Porosity. *Social Studies of Science, 44*(5), 680–700.

Calvert, J., & Fujimura, J. (2011). Calculating Life? Duelling Discourses in Interdisciplinary Systems Biology. *Studies in History and Philosophy of Biological and Biomedical Sciences, 42*, 155–163.

Collins, H. (2010). *Tacit and Explicit Knowledge*. Chicago: University of Chicago Press.

Collins, F. (2011). Reengineering Translational Science: The Time Is Right. *Science Translational Medicine, 3*(90).

D'Argenio, V. (2018). The High-Throughput Analyses Era: Are We Ready for the Data Struggle? *High-Throughput, 7*(1), 8–10.

Doing, P. (2011). Tacit Knowledge. Discovery by or Topic for Science Studies? *Social Studies of Science, 41*(2), 301–306.

Drolet, B., & Lorenzi, N. (2011). Translational Research: Understanding the Continuum from Bench to Bedside. *Translational Research, 157*(1), 1–6.

Erickson, M. (2016). *Science, Culture and Society* (2nd ed.). Cambridge: Polity Press.

Fleck, L. (1935). *Genesis and the Development of a Scientific Fact*. Chicago: University of Chicago Press.

Friese, C. (2013). Realizing Potential in Translational Medicine: The Uncanny Emergence of Care as Science. *Current Anthropology, 54*(S7), S129–S138.

Harrington, J., & Hauskeller, C. (2014). Translational Research: An Imperative Shaping the Spaces in Biomedicine. *Technoscienza, 5*(1), 191–201.

Horrobin, D. (2003). Modern Biomedical Research: An Internally Self-Consistent Universe with Little Contact with Medical Reality? *Nature Reviews: Drug Discovery, 2*, 151–154.

Jacobs, S. (2006). Models of Scientific Community. *Interdisciplinary Science Reviews, 31*(2), 163–173.

Kastenhofer, K. (2013). Two Sides of the Same Coin? The (Techno)epistemic Cultures of Systems and Synthetic Biology. *Studies in History and Philosophy of Biological and Biomedical Sciences, 44*, 130–140.
Keating, P., & Cambrosio, A. (2003). *Biomedical Platforms: Realigning the Normal and Pathological in Late-Twentieth Century Medicine*. Cambridge, MA: MIT Press.
Kitano, H. (2004). Biological Robustness. *Nature Review Genetics, 59*, 826–837.
Knorr Cetina, K. (1983). The Ethnographic Study of Scientific Work: Towards a Constructionist Interpretation of Science. In K. Knorr Cetina & M. Mulkay (Eds.), *Science Observed: Perspectives on the Social Study of Science* (pp. 125–140). London: Sage.
Knorr Cetina, K. (1999). *Epistemic Cultures: The Cultures of Knowledge Societies*. Cambridge, MA: Harvard University Press.
Knorr Cetina, K. (2005). Culture in Global Knowledge Societies: Knowledge Cultures and Epistemic Cultures. In S. Jacobs & N. Weiss Hanrahan (Eds.), *The Blackwell Companion to the Sociology of Culture* (pp. 65–79). Oxford: Blackwell.
Kuhn, T. (1970). *The Structure of Scientific Revolutions* (2nd ed.). Chicago: Chicago University Press.
van der Laan, A., & Boenink, M. (2015). Beyond Bench and Bedside: Disentangling the Concept of Translational Research. *Health Care Analysis, 23*, 32–49.
Landecker, H. (2007). *Culturing Life*. London: Harvard University Press.
Latour, B. (1987). *Science in Action: How to Follow Scientists and Engineers through Society*. Cambridge, MA: Harvard University Press.
Latour, B. (2005). *Reassembling the Social: An Introduction to Actor-Network-Theory*. Oxford: Oxford University Press.
Latour, B., & Woolgar, S. (1979). *Laboratory Life: The Construction of Scientific Facts*. Princeton, NJ: Princeton University Press.
Law, J. (1992). *Notes on the Theory of the Actor Network: Ordering, Strategy and Heterogeneity*. Centre for Science Studies, Lancaster University, Lancaster.
Law, J. (2002). *Aircraft Stories: Decentering the Object in Technoscience*. Durham, NC and London: Duke University Press.
Levin, N. (2014). What's Being Translated in Translational Research? *Technoscienza, 5*(1), 91–113.
Polanyi, M. (1958). *Personal Knowledge: Towards a Post-Critical Philosophy*. Chicago: Chicago University Press.
Polanyi, M. (1985). *Implizites Wissen [1966]*. Frankfurt am Main: Suhrkamp.
Sismondo, S. (2010). *An Introduction to Science and Technology Studies* (2nd ed.). Chichester: Wiley-Blackwell.

The 'Gaze' of the Neurosciences 4

Abstract

This chapter begins by outlining a history of the development of the cognitive neurosciences in its journey from being an esoteric laboratory-based field of research to the spreading of its influence within psychiatry and beyond into the social and cultural spheres. The chapter examines the impact of neuro-imaging technology in revolutionising the ability of scientists to create visual representations of the working of the human brain. It explores these processes utilising the notion of the 'gaze' and the process of 'black-boxing'. This is followed by a discussion of the reasons why the brain sciences now pose a significant challenge to the psychological model of mental health. The chapter concludes by examining autism spectrum disorder as a case study of neuropsychiatric intervention.

Introduction

This chapter and the one that follows examine developments in the field of the cognitive neurosciences over the past half-century. They will assess the ways in which research into the functional pathways of the brain led onto innovative developments in imaging technology, which then opened up the possibilities for the field to expand in many new directions. The drivers of social behaviour and mental health once the preserve of psychology have arguably now been reconceptualised in neurological terms. At the most uncompromising end of this radical re-imaging of the role of neuroscientific analysis is the view, 'that our brains hold the key to whom we are' (Rose and Abi-Rached 2013: 1).

The assessment of the neurosciences in society has been separated into two chapters to give due prominence to the epistemological differences that exist between realist and social constructionist forms of analysis. These approaches are not

I. Crinson, *The Biomedical Sciences in Society*,
https://doi.org/10.1007/978-981-15-9523-3_4

mutually exclusive, and to utilise a phrase drawn from the study of aerodynamics, each methodology represents a different 'angle of attack' on the subject matter. An appreciation of the contribution of both traditions of social analysis ultimately results in a more nuanced and critical assessment of the social application of cognitive neuroscience research.

This chapter examines the impact of neuro-imaging technology in revolutionising the ability of neuroscientists to create visual representations of the working of the human brain. The apparent ability of these technological developments to localise complex cognitive processes is discussed in terms of the concept of the 'clinical gaze'. The discussion then moves onto an examination of the process of 'black-boxing' and its consequences for the science. The chapter continues with a discussion of the challenges that neuroscience now sets to the traditional psychological conceptualisation of mental illness as a disorder of the mind or as disturbances of the psyche. And, it concludes with two case studies of the 'hope' and the 'uncertainty' that have accompanied the application of the neuroscience in seeking to further the understanding, and potentially the treatment, of autism spectrum disorder.

The Emergent Field of Cognitive Neuroscience

The roots of modern cognitive neuroscience lie in what has been termed the 'cognitive turn' in psychology that can be traced back to the late 1950s. This was the moment when behaviourism, the previously dominant paradigm in psychology, began its gradual slide to the margins of the discipline. It was replaced by a new way of thinking about information processing within the brain, cognitive capacity, and function.

Behaviourism as a theory of human learning had been predicated on the understanding that all learnt behaviours (animal and human) were reactive, the outcome of 'operant conditioning' (learning as a process of associating a stimulus with reward or with punishment) that occurred as a consequence of interactions with the external environment. Behaviourist psychological research focused on stimulating and then observing the outward behaviour of animals, think Pavlov and his dogs and Skinner and his boxes for testing the operant conditioning of rats and pigeons. Behaviour was perceived as the only objective way of understanding the process of learning, rejecting explanations involved active internal processes. The critique of the predictive failings of behaviourism led onto the development of what some termed 'cognitive studies', and others 'information processing psychology', and finally in the early 1970s, 'cognitive science' (Miller 2003: 142). The new cognitive sciences drew upon ideas and concepts from the pre-existing fields of linguistics, cognitive psychology, and anthropology; these were combined with new ways of thinking about information processing emanating from the emerging fields of the neurosciences and computer science. This 'revolution' in thinking was predicated on the possibility that the brain was an information processing control computer developed through processes of evolution and natural selection.

At the same time, what were then referred to as the 'brain sciences' were also responding to the challenges of cognitive science. These brain sciences then became sub-divided into 'behavioural neuroscience' (also termed 'physiological psychology') and 'systems neuroscience', formed out of the interactions between physiology, anatomy, and psychology. While behavioural neuroscience focused on brain–behaviour relations, systems neuroscience was concerned primarily with the neural circuits involved in specific brain structures such as the hippocampus. The primary sources of evidence for both sub-disciplines remained animal studies. Hence, the major transmission route for the new information-processing conception of human mental processes emanated not from the traditional brain sciences as such, but from the new theoretical frameworks being developed within the clinical field of cognitive psychology (Cooper and Shallice 2010: 399).

From its early beginnings therefore, cognitive neuroscience was forged as an interdisciplinary field combining analysis at many different levels, cellular, molecular, anatomical, physiological, and behavioural. It was recognised that breakthroughs in understanding neural processes would only be achieved by a synthesis of these diverse methodologies, a common intellectual space for disciplines to interact. Nevertheless, in the intervening years since the field of cognitive neuroscience first emerged, one distinctive vision of the brain has come to take on precedence in the field. This is the position that the mental functions of human perception, cognition, emotion, and volition can in principle all be accounted for by processes operating at the molecular level, constituting a biological substrate to cognitive neuroscience. The field of cognitive neuroscience has developed and expanded through a series of discontinuous events, but today it has reached the stage where it is able to confidently delineate its epistemic concerns. To offer one example, the Center for Cognitive Neuroscience at the University of Pennsylvania, one of many academic centres of neuroscience research that now exist throughout the globe, sets out its mission to understand the neural bases of human thought in terms of the following:

> *Our current research addresses the central problems of cognitive neuroscience, including perception, attention, learning, memory, language, decision-making, emotion and development. Our methods are equally diverse, and include functional neuroimaging, behavioral testing of neurological and psychiatric patients, transcranial and direct current magnetic stimulation, scalp-recorded event-related potentials, intracranial recording, computational modeling, candidate gene studies and pharmacologic manipulations of cognitive processes.* (http://ccn.upenn.edu/, accessed Sept 2019)

An Introduction to Medical Perception and the 'Clinical Gaze'

A key analytical concept drawn upon by social constructionists in conceptualising the ways in which clinicians engage in the process of constructing the nature of illness, whether physical or mental, is that of the 'clinical gaze'. This concept was first utilised by Michel Foucault in his classic text, *The Birth of the Clinic* published in 1973, which sets out his particular historical reading or 'archaeology' of the development of modern medicine. Foucault's goal was to assess 'the conditions of possibility' for doctors in the early nineteenth century to instigate a radically new way of perceiving the illness experienced by their patients.

The early nineteenth century was the period during which clinical medicine was becoming a professionalised field of expertise, yet the clinical understanding of illness still remained a two-dimensional process. Signs of disease were looked for in exterior tissues of patients, but doctors were crucially reliant on listening to the patient's own accounts of their malady. But developments in optical instrumentation and the invention of the stethoscope were able to facilitate the construction of a new three-dimensional view of the body. That is, the ability to 'see' the internal organs and to so define 'normality' in terms of the absence of pathology. An approach facilitated by 'an increasing fidelity to what can be revealed by sense-perceptible data' (Foucault 1973: 136). This ability to 'gaze', to assess the internal processes of the living human body, also enabled early modern medicine to develop textbook categorisations of disease. However, deploying the 'gaze' led onto an objectification of patients, denying a role for their own accounts of illness in the process of medical diagnosis. Within Foucault's work, the clinical gaze is therefore 'cast as monological and reductive, rather than dialogical and exploratory' (Bleakley and Bligh 2009: 370). As we shall see later in this chapter, the application of brain-imaging technologies in the twenty-first century has transformed this gaze from a literal to a simulated reading of the patient (Bleakley and Bligh 2009: 376). On this last point, it should be noted that Foucault's notion of the clinical gaze constitutes a qualitatively different analytical viewpoint from that of later ANT studies of representations of disease, discussed below.

Despite the fact that both positions sharing a common anti-realist philosophy, Foucault's focus is on the relationship between knowledge and power in the construction of a professional 'discourse' able to 'configure' and 'localise' the classification of disease. In *The Birth of the Clinic* (1973), Foucault describes power in relation to the shaping of these parameters of physical disease through the gaze of the emergent profession of medicine, while in his *Madness and Civilisation* (1967/1989), he analyses the construction of madness as illness through the gaze of the emergent profession of psychiatry (discussed below). For Foucault, power is inseparably linked to the application of knowledge (what he termed 'knowledge/power'), and as such he consistently poses the question of in whose interests is this power exercised? In contrast, ANT studies present the construction of disease events as an outcome of a joint enterprise or network involving both human (scientists and professionals) and non-human (technologies, ideas) actors. Bruno Latour, one of the leading figures in ANT, strongly asserts that '(W)e need to get rid of all categories like those of power, knowledge, profit or capital, because they divide up a cloth that we want seamless in order to study it as we choose' (1987: 223).

The Path from Laboratory-Based Research to Clinical Interventions

In discussing the expansion of the neurosciences in the twenty-first century in their book, *Neuro: The New Brain Sciences and the Management of the Mind*, Nick Rose and Joelle Abe-Rached (2013) have drawn attention to what they describe as four 'transactional points' in the neuroscience's journey from an esoteric field of research to the spreading of its influence to the clinical field of psychiatry and increasingly beyond into the social and cultural spheres.

Their first 'transactional point' was the development of the field of psychopharmacology. Historically, drug interventions for mental illness were given only to patients within the walls of psychiatric hospitals, but over time as these drugs were seen to be relatively effective and safe so they began to be prescribed by GP's in primary care to individuals living with incapacitating depressive forms of illness. The origins of psychopharmacology as a clinical field derive from research conducted in the 1950s (almost all using animal models) from which emerged the view that states of mental disorder could and should be understood in terms of disruptions of neuromolecular processes. These were identified as pathologies of neurotransmission, hence the promotion of the 'monamine hypothesis' as an explanation for the causes of depression and the 'dopamine hypothesis' in relation to schizophrenia. These theories were the first significant representation of a conceptual and chemical linkage between mental illness and neurotransmitters. Most importantly, this new field of research brought together for the first time the neurobiological research community, pharmaceutical companies, and the profession of psychiatry. However, over the subsequent decades both hypotheses and associated chemical treatments proved to be less than efficacious and are now often conceptualised as the 'founding myths' of psychopharmacology.

The second transactional point occurred at the end of the twentieth century with the emergence of the field of research known as 'neurogenomics'. The latter combines neurobiology and genomics to examine how the human genome contributes to the evolution, development, structure, and function of the nervous system. While genetic explanations of mental disorders had existed since the 1950s (and can be traced back further to the eugenics movement of the early part of the twentieth century—see Chap. 7 for an outline), by the late 1980s claims were being made for the potential of discovering a single 'gene for' a whole list of mental health conditions, including schizophrenia and depression. It was the completion of the sequencing of the human genome at the beginning of this century that finally enabled radical developments in the genomic understanding of mental functioning to occur. Genomics focuses at levels of variation in single bases of DNA sequences rather than whole genes, and the ways in which small variations in the sequence might affect the nature of the protein synthesised or activities of the particular enzyme. The goal for neurogenomics was not only to elucidate the genomic bases of neurological disease, but also to achieve the translational goals of developing disease-modifying and preventive therapies. Unfortunately, these developments have not been forthcoming as anticipated. The majority of neurological diseases are sporadic without any obvious familial or genetic occurrence, and the molecular bases of neurological diseases, particularly neurodegenerative diseases, largely remain unknown (Tsuji 2013).

The third translational point identified by Rose and Abi-Rached (2013) is the recognition of brain plasticity. Embracing the notion of plasticity in brain structure represents a crucial conceptual shift from the view that cognitive capacity is inscribed by inherited genes at conception towards a much more dynamic and fluid understanding of the development of neural architecture occurring over a life course. The notion of plasticity originally derived from clinical research that demonstrated that it was not just at the level of the synapse that 'rewiring' could occur after a brain or spinal injury but that the process of neurogenesis was possible throughout adult life. This new thinking was supported by developments in epigenetics and the understanding of the influence of the environment at the level of molecular processes of the genome (discussed in Chap. 7). For example, that early maternal behaviour (the findings again deriving from animal research) could shape the neural development of babies, with implications for their behaviour over a whole lifetime.

The fourth translational point is seen as the exponential developments that have occurred in neuro-imaging, facilitated by the development of powerful computer technologies that first became available for research purposes in the 1990s. This technology has resulted in the production of not only clear images of the structure of the brain, but its apparent functioning in real time: '(A)s these technologies became more widely available to researchers, thousands of papers were published claiming to identify the neural correlates of every human mental state from love to hate' (Rose and Abi-Rached 2013: 13).

We now move onto a more detailed analysis of the claims for neuro-imaging as enhancing our understanding of the functioning of the human brain. This discussion focuses on STS accounts of modes of representation.

Neuro-Imaging Research: Localisation, Representation, and 'Black Boxes'

> *(T)he most ubiquitous icon of neuroscientific power today appears to be the brain scan. Often compelling, these evocative representations of cerebral matter are ciphers over which a variety of professionals and publics have come to lay their own understandings of personhood.* (Pickersgill 2013: 326)

The primary scientific methodology for understanding the brain up until the late nineteenth century was the systematic global observation of individuals exteriorising their emotions, but over time an alternative approach gained traction. This was represented in the shift from the global to a localised view of the brain as an internally differentiated organ. An early and well-known example of this new understanding was Broca's work in the 1850s on speech loss, which was able to localise the speech centre of the brain in the left frontal lobe of the brain. Much of this early research was undertaken with animals, artificially creating lesions in specific areas of the brain and studying their consequences. The nerve cell was first isolated and described by Otto Deiters in 1865, and subsequent research focused on the question of whether nerve cells formed a continuous network or were contiguous (sharing a border, not touching). This work eventually led on to the development of the technique of nerve cell staining which opened up the brain to early forms of scientific representation. In the early twentieth century, research into the functional architecture of the brain was inadvertently aided by the brain trauma experienced by thousands of soldiers during the First World War. These case studies were constructed on the basis that reverse mapping was a viable technique for developing an understanding of function, the linking of known damage to a particular part of the brain to observed disruption of normal functioning. Yet the study of the links between mental disorders and particular neural structures could not be translated into any viable clinical interventions for most of the twentieth century. Methods such as cortical stimulation by surgical probe in the 1950s further contributed to the mapping of cerebral localised structures and their apparent functions, but less intrusive methods were required to further this vision.

Almost certainly, the single most influential advance in the neuroscientific understanding of cognitive processes was the development of what is colloquially referred to as 'brain scanning', more accurately, neuro-imaging techniques and methodologies. These technologies were initially developed as clinical diagnostic technologies to image internal organs (not exclusively the brain), for example, providing information about whether macroscopic lesions were present or not in the brain of patients. Only later were scanning technologies taken up as 'inscription devices' for research purposes and used to provide information not about lesions but about brain function. These early scanning technologies, which included computerised tomography (CT) and magnetic resonance imaging (MRI), were very useful for detecting structural abnormalities but were not able to provide images of what the living brain was doing. In the late 1980s positron emission tomography (PET) was first used to measure differences in regional cerebral blood flow (rCBF) using radiotracers. These imaging technologies were premised upon the assumption that areas of high radioactivity were associated with increased cognitive information processing. Neuroscientists argued that rCBF changes in identified brain regions mirrored their functioning when undertaking cognitive tasks. A second imaging technique, functional magnetic resonance imaging (fMRI), was developed in the early 1990s. This was utilised to overcome some of the problems arising from the dependence on radioactivity levels as a proxy measure for cognitive activity. The development of fMRI was the culmination of the increasing sophistication of MRI algorithms, it became possible to take successive images and link them together in order to capture as many as hundred plus frames per second. A second important development was the search for a suitable tissue that could be imaged and linked to functional activity. That tissue was blood, which had the added advantage of possessing magnetic properties. Interestingly, the correlation of blood flow with increased blood activity has had a long antecedence going back to nineteenth-century science.

Dumit (2014) has identified four stages in the design and application of neuroimaging technologies for research purposes and the ways in which this engineering process has incorporated a number of implicit social assumptions. While Dumit's work focuses on the development of PET brain scanning technologies, at the general level of analysis, his conclusions apply just as much to the design of fMRI technologies. The first stage is the devising of the experimental design, which involves choosing the research participants, defining their condition (normal/pathological), unambiguously specifying the tasks they are to carry out in the scanner, and controlling their prior states. The second stage involves managing the technical process of measuring brain activity, the compiling of activity data, and algorithmically reconstructing a three-dimensional map. The third stage is all about making the data comparable. This involves transforming, warping, and stretching the data for each individual to fit a standard anatomical atlas of brain space. The final stage involves making the data presentable; this is achieved through the process of colouring, contrasting, and production of the images using now standardised software.

To return to the first and second phases of the experimental process, it is worth saying a little bit more about a key aspect of this process known as 'cognitive subtraction'. The Italian neuroscientists Paolo Legrenzi and Carlo Umiltà (2011) have described the steps involved in utilising this experimental methodology. First it requires a comparison of two conditions or brain states that are presumed to differ in only one discrete feature. The next step is to identify a control task that involves all the functions of the experimental task with the exception of those processes whose neural bases are the focus of the experiment itself (the independent variable). The person participating in the experiment is asked to perform both tasks in succession, and while each task is being carried out, the neuro-imaging technology measures the activation of very small regions of the brain (3 mm cubes) known as 'voxels' (which can contain over a million neurons each), then an 'activation vector' is obtained for both tasks. The level of activation obtained in the control task is subtracted voxel by voxel from that obtained in the experimental task. This in theory provides a non-zero result for those voxels which correspond to the cerebral areas that become active during the experimental task (Lagrenzi and Umiltà 2011: 23–24). The experimental process therefore relies on 'the assumption of "pure insertion"—the notion that a single cognitive process can be inserted into a task without affecting the remaining processes, or that there are no interactions among the cognitive components of a task' (Harrison and Pentalis 2010). However in practice, the human brain experiences simultaneous activation of multiple areas in the course of everyday activity and interaction. This is a big problem for neuro-imaging research, as activation can be influenced by chance factors that cannot be controlled for by the experimenter. As a consequence, the 'chance probability' associated with the result of the subtraction has to be calculated for each of the million plus voxels; an exceedingly difficult task. So when neuroscientists assert that a particular localised area is delegated for a specific function, or the cause of a specific psychological effect, what in fact is being represented 'is the result of a graphic device which transforms chance probability into colour and is then superimposed on a drawing of the brain' (Legrenzi and Umiltà 2011: 26).

The conversion of data into arbitrary colours in brain images has undoubtedly played an important role in their appeal to the public. But the use of colour to visually highlight areas of activity or inactivity in 'regions of interest' can make quite small differences in the data appear large and quite stark. The colour red is usually allocated to areas that show increases in activity, from pale pink indicating just about statistically significant activity to bright scarlet allocated to the most significant. Blue is allocated to decreases in activity, again ranging from pale to bright. Areas where there are no changes are not coloured. Hence, the 'overwhelming impression that you are looking at the equivalent of a photograph of a living, thinking human brain, beautifully colour-coded to show where "thoughts" were coming from and seeming to provide irrefutable evidence of the "mindreading" power of neuro-imagers' (Rippon 2019: 74). Despite these methodological concerns, the neuroscience assertion of the experimental validity of neuro-imaging technology marks a significant shift towards what has been described as both the 'biologisation' and 'digitalisation' of human behavioural and psychological processes. This is where '(T)he discrete, mapped-out bright bits seem to provide visual proof for the existence of material substrates of behavioural mechanisms, and for the claim that the basis of the mind is biological' (de Rijcke and Beaulieu 2014: 131).

The refinements in fMRI analysis and experimental design are seen in popular discourse to have opened up the interior processes of the living and dynamic brain and leading onto the claim that such technologies render the mind as 'visible'. This is the motivation for STS researchers to question the ontological claims of neuroscientists when they make claims about the tractability of brain processes (Coopmans et al. 2014: 4). Three assumptions are seen as underpinning the now widespread assimilation of neuro-imaging technologies in neuroscience research as visual representations of brain processes: (1) the localisation of brain processes, (2) the neutrality of the laboratory, and (3) the design of technologies. Each of these assumptions will be examined in detail below.

As we have already seen, localisation is a key organising principle in cognitive neuroscience. It assumes a hard-wired connection of neurons such that specific mental processes are assigned to specified regions of the brain in all 'normal' human beings. The ontological assumption that underpins localisation can be seen as a reflective of the modular structural-function relationships to be found generally within the biomedical sciences. In practice, 'many cognitive processes may be distinguished not by activity in specific regions but by patterns of activity across regions, (so) there is reason for caution regarding many of the inferences that have been drawn by highly modular approaches' (Poldrack 2008, cited in Rose and Abe-Rached 2013: 76). Localisation cannot also easily account for the process of neuroplasticity, also discussed above, as a key feature of learning and memory. Although the neurobiological basis of synaptic plasticity is now well established, the system-level dynamics of this process remain unclear (Assaf 2018).

The second assumption concerns the physical space of the laboratory or clinic in which the scanning of experimental human subjects takes place. This is often assumed to be a neutral factor, but there is strong evidence that the settings of research play an important role in influencing the generation of imaging data. Given that neuro-imaging research is often focused on 'normal' functioning of the brain, the scanning facility in which subjects are asked to perform tasks that mimic activity in the social world, while lying down in a noisy and confining scanning machine, is anything but a normal situation. This issue draws attention to the social relations found in the research facility and the impact they have on the mental processes of the scanned individual.

The third and final assumption relates to the design and the application of neuro-imaging technologies and their standardised software packages. STS analysis, as we have previously seen, is concerned to assess the processes by which scientists construct their knowledge claims, and in such analyses, the notion of the 'black box' is often drawn upon as an explanatory metaphor. As applied more generally in science, the 'black box' usually depicts an unknown or uncertain system where only the inputs and outputs are known. But within STS research, the term is utilised in a rather different way. Here it is used to describe the process by which a scientific object becomes 'stabilised' over time. At first this object of research (e.g., some aspect of brain function) might be simply a list of attributes, then a description of experimental data, but overtime these attributes may no longer be questioned and so become stabilised as 'facts'. The application of such attributes in other experimental research settings further reinforce these stabilising facts, which are then published within scientific papers, further stabilising the object over a wide range of scientific actors (Deschauer 2011: 35). Eventually the 'facts' appear to be the attributes of the scientific object in question. Bruno Latour explains the process of 'black-boxing' as follows: '(T)he way scientific and technical work is made invisible by its own success. When a machine runs efficiently, when a matter of fact is settled, one need focus only on its inputs and outputs and not on its internal complexity. Thus, paradoxically, the more science and technology succeed, the more opaque and obscure they become' (Latour 1999: 304).

Potential ontological errors (neuroscience assumptions about the whole range of processes involved in the functioning of the brain) may arise when neuro-imaging is driven by 'the technically sweet possibilities of reverse engineering the brain that arise from new and improved technologies, rather than by scientific questions aimed at teasing apart different cognitive theories or extending our cognitive understanding of specific processes' (Cooper and Shallice 2010: 403). Or to put it more bluntly, technology alone, even where it appears to measure neural activity, 'cannot enable the *gaze* to bridge the gap between molecules and mental states' (Rose 1986: 92).

Constructing Mental Disorders: From Psychiatry to Neuroscience

Psychological conceptions of the mind constituted the basis for the explanation of human behaviour for virtually the whole of the twentieth century. Psychology shaped societal reactions to and the treatment of mental illness (via the clinical profession of psychiatry), it influenced child-rearing and educational initiatives, as well as providing a commentary on many other aspects of social life. But today, the cognitive neuroscience presents a significant challenge to this particular understanding of behaviour and mental health.

A particularly influential text that has assessed the historical construction of mental illness alongside the evolving power of the profession of psychiatry is another of Michel Foucault publications; this one is entitled *Madness and Civilization* (1967/1989) given the subtitle 'A History of Madness in an Age of Reason'. This is a historical account of the imposition of a rationality that led to the social exclusion and incarceration within asylums of a social group deemed as 'unreasonable'. The designation of madness as psychiatric illness by the emergent profession of psychiatry in the early nineteenth century was 'not a discovery of an objective truth but a result of the convergence of internment and medicine' (Cousins and Hussain 1984: 139). As Foucault describes it, the imposition of the new psychiatric gaze meant that 'the victim of mental illness is entirely alienated in the real person of his doctor, the doctor dissipates the reality of the mental illness in the critical concept of madness' (Foucault 1967/1989: 86). Yet in the nineteenth century, the new psychiatric understanding of mental illness remained largely at the level of surface impressions, predicated on a belief that emotions were manifested in visual expressions. This was not so far removed from the pseudo-science of phrenology that had also begun to focus on the physiognomy of madness in the early nineteenth century, developing a taxonomy based on skull shape and facial appearance. By the mid-nineteenth century, the development of photographic images of asylum inmates further contributed to this exteriority of madness.

The high point of visualising mental distress through the comportment of the body and expressions of the face came at the end of the nineteenth century, in work of Jean-Martin Charcot, an eminent French professor of neurology and anatomical pathology. Charcot is often described as the father of modern-day neurology (he was the first clinician to identify multiple sclerosis), and in his clinical teaching to students at the Salpêtrière hospital in Paris, he would often mimic the clinical signs of certain diseases to his students—the asymmetry of the face in facial paralysis, the rigidity of Parkinson's disease, and various types of tics, spasms, postures, and various unusual gaits. He stressed the importance of close observation and would subject his patients to a slow, systematic scrutiny for several minutes without saying a word. Charcot also utilised the concept of brain localisation, leading his students from one salient point of the case to another (Jay 2000: 10). He was to drew on this systematic approach to undertake the first significant classification or 'nosology' of neurological disease. Interestingly, one of Charcot's star pupils was Sigmund Freud, who was later to turn away from these images of mental illness and to listen to his patients talk about their distress, a very different form of representation of the 'unconscious mind'.

Over the course of twentieth century, psychiatry as a profession attempted to follow the approach of physical medicine in developing a standardised system for the classification of disease. The first classificatory system known as the 'International List of Causes of Death' had been adopted by the International Statistical Institute in 1893. Following the post-war establishment of the World Health Organisation (WHO), it was this international body that took on the responsibility of revising and updating the list, changing the title, and publishing the 6th Edition of the 'International Classification of Diseases' in 1948 (ICD-6). The current iteration, ICD-11, was released in 2018. The psychiatric medicine equivalent of the ICD was first published by the American Psychiatric Association in 1952 and was termed the 'Diagnostic and Statistical Manual' (DSM) for mental disorders. The DSM-IV published in 1994 introduced for the first time the criterion of 'clinical significance' in order to avoid the false-positive diagnoses that arose from overly inclusive classifications of disorders in previous editions of the DSM (DSM-II in 1968; DSM-III in 1980). However, these cautions did not prevent the new classificatory system from being questioned by one group of psychiatrists who concluded that '(a)bout half of Americans will meet the criteria for a DSM-IV disorder sometime in their life, with first onset usually in childhood or adolescence' (Kessler et al. 2005—cited in Rose and Abi-Rached 2013: 125). False-positive diagnoses continued to arise because the diagnostic criteria of the DSM did not take account of individual context and so did not adequately discriminate between 'normal' responses to stressful life events, such as grief, sadness, and anxiety, and those pathological conditions that require psychiatric intervention.

The difficulties faced by the profession of psychiatry in attempting to emulate the consistency of diagnosis and efficacy in the clinical management of physical disease opened the door to an alternative neuromolecular conceptualisation of mental distress and social behaviour. In Rose and Abi-Rached's (2013) constructivist account, the neuropsychological understanding of mental distress was only able to begin to displace the psychology of the mind and effect change in practice when two historical binary boundaries had been overcome or at least blurred. These binaries constituted the foundation on which the knowledge base of psychiatry had been successfully constructed in the twentieth century.

The first of these binary boundaries that was successfully overcome was the Cartesian mind-body 'split'. The ability to separate out disorders that were seen to arise from identifiable organic lesions in the brain, and those disturbances of mental functioning that had no known organic basis, deriving from personal biographies and other social experiences, was crucial to the development of psychiatry in the late nineteenth century. In cognitive neuroscience, there is no need to perpetuate this dualism, as all disorders are seen to have a potentially identifiable neural basis (Rose and Abi-Rached 2013: 38). The second binary is that drawn between 'states' and 'traits', from which arose the distinction drawn between psychiatry and psychology. 'States' being intermittent periods of illness or distress, when an individual who was previously well becomes depressed but with treatment is able to return to an optimal state of normality. The focus on these 'abnormal states' has been the preserve of psychiatry and its interventions. 'Traits' are attributes that an individual is said to have been born with personality disorders, melancholia, and so on. These character traits could not be treated but only assessed and managed. This distinction constituted the basis for the development of psychology as an academic discipline. But if traits and states are seen to be simply variations of the same neuromolecular set of processes, then this distinction disappears (Rose and Abi-Rached 2013: 46).

Cognitive neuroscience appears to settle the uncertainty of psychiatric diagnosis by identifying the underlying neural processes of mental illness. Its attraction for patient groups is the possibility of no longer equating mental illness with personal or parental responsibility, so making it difficult to sustain social stigma and blame. The possibilities for neuropsychiatric-based interventions for mental illness lie with three interlinked developments in the field: (1) The use of identifiable genetic markers and brain pattern imaging in order to provide a neurobiological basis for psychiatric classification, so furthering the understanding of the aetiology of mental disorder, which in turn forms the basis for (2) an effective screening programme and (3) the development of effective treatments targeting the neurobiological basis of mental disorders.

The actuality of neuropsychiatric approaches to the identification and treatment of mental ill-health has though been questioned. In part, this is because the process of establishing phenotypes (see Glossary) of mental disorder is problematic given that similar symptoms can result from different combinations of genetic risk factors. At the same time, the same genetic variant may be associated with multiple DSM diagnoses. Additionally, there are many environmental and other random events that contribute to mental illness not predicated on whole genomic make-up. This problem of identifying phenotypes is one of the reasons why Genome-Wide Association Studies (see Glossary) often fail in psychiatry. Despite their apparent complexity, GWAS are too reductionist when applied to mental disorder. Any attempt to identify a particular 'gene for' a particular psychiatric disorder has to resolve the dilemma of genes being essentially pleiotropic (a single gene may produce a number of effects, i.e., two or more seemingly unrelated phenotypic traits). Note: The application of GWAS within the clinical field of pharmacogenomics is discussed in detail in Chap. 6.

Hope and Uncertainty: Neuroscience and the Case of Autism Spectrum Disorder

As we have seen, the neurosciences and its associated research technologies such as neuro-imaging now fulfil an integral role in epistemologically privileging the brain as the source of psychopathology. That is, neuroscience-based explanations of behavioural and cognitive disorders are today frequently perceived as being more legitimate than other forms of explanation, even when it 'adds nothing substantial to the explanation' (Bertorelli 2016: 505). The majority of neuroscientists are realistic about the challenges they face in translating laboratory-acquired knowledge into effective treatments for various disorders. However, there remains the temptation for some to be less than critical, given the incentives of large-scale funding from pharmaceutical companies and government research agencies. There is additionally the pressure of social expectations, fuelled by the 'promissory discourses' of neuroscience, to develop innovative interventions for mental illness and developmental disorders. Social scientists working within the tradition of STS have sought to explore these social expectations of hope linked to the promise of the neurosciences. These developments will be discussed below in relation to autism spectrum disorder (ASD) research.

There has been a significant increase in the reported prevalence of ASD in the last two decades, and as such, the condition has emerged as an issue of growing social concern. ASD is a complex neurodevelopmental spectrum disorder without a clear-cut specificity, as is implied from the use of the terms 'spectrum' and 'disorder'. It is a condition that is also characterised by a high degree of uncertainty and contestation, with important implications for all key participants in the management of the condition, including the parents of children diagnosed with ADH, neuroscientists, and clinical professionals. Over time there have been significant changes made in the classificatory diagnostic criteria for the condition found within the DSM, as well the more commonly used (in the UK) ICD. The DSM-V lists two areas of relevance to the diagnosis of this condition: '(P)ersistent deficits in social communication and social interaction across multiple contexts' and 'restricted, repetitive patterns of behavior, interests, or activities' (APA 2013). It lists symptoms as being 'present in the early developmental period but that these may not become fully manifest until social demands exceed limited capacities, or may be masked by learned strategies in later life' (APA 2013). The diagnostic criteria set out three distinct severity levels for ASD, although some latitude is allowed for individual variation in both core and non-ASD symptoms. It should be noted that neuro-imaging is not currently a component of the diagnostic process for ASD in the UK (NHS 2017), but it is used extensively in research conducted into ASD, discussed below.

Based on qualitative research interviews, and drawing upon a 'sociology of expectations' framework (see Text Box 2 in Chap. 6), Des Fitzgerald (2014) has written an insightful STS paper exploring the views of UK-based neuroscientists working within the AST research field. His findings pointing to the emergence of what he terms a 'discourse of ambiguity' surrounding ASD research. This 'discourse' is seen to reflect the fact that ASD research draws on both structural and functional neuro-imaging technologies that lack the specificity of an identifiable and convincing brain-based biomarker for the condition, one that can be replicated across time or research site. This uncertainty has meant that there is a continuing reliance on behavioural measures of ASD and the ability of skilled clinical professionals to identify the presence of the condition within individuals. At the same time, and somewhat ironically, autism continues to retain an identity as a genetic disorder of the brain. This leaves neuroscientists both unable to ignore the condition's lack of specificity, but acknowledging the legitimate desire of parents and clinicians alike, for a neurogenetic basis to the disorder to be identified. Fitzgerald argues that in the face of this uncertainty, neuroscientists attempt to manage their own research expectations through constructing a narrative path of both 'promise and unease through this ambivalent dynamic' (Fitzgerald 2014: 246).

Fitzgerald also found that the neuroscientists acknowledged the ambiguous nature of ASD as a neurological, genetic, or diagnostic object, while at the same time holding positive views about identifying differences in neurological anatomy between autistic and 'typically developing' people. The latter approach is seen to be a potential research pathway for future effective neurological interventions at an early age. One of the neuropsychiatrists interviewed in the study demonstrated this hope by comparing a future scenario in which autism would be as instantly diagnosable as a heart attack. This would be ASD research understood in terms of a sociology of expectations, where 'the loose promise of neurological diagnosis and therapy in the future becomes the ground on which large-scale projects are enacted in the present' (Fitzgerald 2014: 248). But Fitzgerald also found a 'strong current of unease and disappointment' among many of the neuroscientists that served to move their narratives away from high expectations about their ASD research: '(T)hey consistently drew my attention to the problem of false positives, the distance between what their methods measured and what they purported to measure, the degree to which neuroimaging simply replicates what is already known through other means; and even the basic inadequacy of brain-imaging to mental phenomena in the first place' (Fitzgerald 2014: 251). Fitzgerald concludes his assessment of these 'low expectancy' outcomes as follows: '(N)eurobiological autism research thus does not progress, even in its own self-narration, in an obviously linear fashion. Instead it works more delicately through the zone of ambiguity and presence that surrounds the biological and social hinterland of autism' (Fitzgerald 2014: 252).

On a similar theme of uncertainty in the neuro-management of ASD, but this time focused on interviews with child and adolescent psychiatrists rather than neuroscientists, Bertorelli's (2016) qualitative study examines 'hope' ('the extent to which neuro-imaging could positively influence understandings of ASD') and 'doubt' ('the extent to which technologies are limited and limiting') among researchers in this field (2016: 509). The outcomes of the interviews point to the existence of a discourse of 'ambivalence' (similar to Fitzgerald's notion of 'low expectancy', but more nuanced) held by these psychiatrists about the consequences of over-relying on the neuroscientific 'gaze' that is built into neuro-imagining technologies. This ambivalence did not represent a rejection of neuro-imaging as a research tool per se, but rather reflected a long-standing tension between behavioural and biopsychiatric approaches, not just in the management of ASD but within the wider clinical field of psychiatry.

In Bertorelli's study, the 'hope' side of ambivalence was directed towards the role of neuro-imaging research as providing evidence for the biological basis of ASD, so debunking the myth of a routine vaccination causation perpetrated in the now discredited research of Andrew Wakefield in the late 1990s (Dyer 2010). Neuro-imaging was also seen to have a promising role in overcoming the heterogeneity of ASD symptoms, which can lead to similar behavioural presentations between two individuals not being connected to the same disorder, so increasing the chances of misdiagnosis (Bertorelli 2016: 511). Neuro-imaging evidence of a biological basis of ASD is also seen as having the potential to dispel parental feelings of guilt and responsibility and by extension 'stigma by association' (see Glossary). The 'doubt' side of the ambivalence expressed by the psychiatrists was directed at the current limitations of the technology used to visualise neural pathways, as well as the perceived reductive biopsychiatric framing of ASD as exclusively a disorder of the brain. As this study points out, the presumed biological basis of ASD does not hold water if it cannot transcend the differences that extend across patient groups, geographies, and cultures (Bertorelli 2016: 515). The 'allure' of neuro-imaging was seen as diverting research attention and funding away from the search for alternative and perhaps more useful social and environmental causative explanations of ASD (Bertorelli 2016: 520).

Both of these case studies of ASD can be described as examples of sociology of 'low expectations' that has its basis in realist social theory rather than the constructivism notion of expectations linked to promissory visions (see Theory Box 6.1 in Chap. 6). The term represents the ways in which scientists attempt to manage disappointing research outcomes in order to sustain their work over the long haul. That is, managing the negative expectations that can arise from attempting to sustain overly ambitious large-scale projects in the face of unanticipated problems. Anticipating problems that might arise during the research process may be conceived as a pessimistic projection but actually constitutes an essential part of a science project. If problems can be anticipated, even if they subsequently do not arise, this remains a necessary undertaking in order to maintain momentum on science research programmes, not being confined to biomedical science (Gardner et al. 2015: 1004).

Concluding Comments

As discussed in Chap. 2, a key (positivist) assumption of science work is that we can measure the world in order to produce data. This data can then be organised to produce meaningful, actionable information, which can be synthesised with scientist's prior experience to produce knowledge of the world. Then, 'in some unspecified way and probably indescribable way, we arrive at a state in which we are able to apply the things we know with the balanced discernment we think of as wisdom' (Greenfield 2017: 210). The underpinning assumption is that scientific 'data' is always objective. Yet even in the contemporary world with highly complex and sophisticated forms of computerised information management, whatever 'we measure and retain with our sensors, as with our bodily sense, is invariably a selection from the far broader array available to us' (Greenfield 2017: 210). In the case of neuro-imaging, this 'selection' is built into the design of the algorithms that drive the fMRI's and PET scanners, from which neuroscientist draw their 'objective' neurobiological constructions of 'brain-based' disorders to 'potential replace traditional psychiatry' (Cohn 2012: 182).

While the neurosciences have undoubtedly made many positive contributions to advancing our knowledge of mental disorder, it is nevertheless unlikely on its own to be able to solve the current diagnostic dilemma's faced by psychiatric medicine. Brain-based diagnosis has had a low predictive validity in terms of prognosis and cannot account for the social and environmental factors that may shape a condition's trajectory over time. It is probably the case that 'no single system could ever bear this weight, but it is certain that one based on the brain alone cannot. At root, the neurobiological project in psychiatry finds its limit in the simple and often repeated fact: mental disorders are problems of persons, not of brains' (Rose and Abi-Rached 2013: 140).

Chapter Summary: Key Points

- *The roots of modern cognitive neuroscience lie in what has been termed the 'cognitive turn' in psychology that can be traced back to the late 1950s.*
- *From its very beginning, cognitive neuroscience was an interdisciplinary field, combining analysis at the cellular, molecular, anatomical, physiological, and behavioural levels.*
- *Four key 'transactional points' in the journey of neuroscience from an esoteric field of research to influence within the social and cultural spheres have been identified.*
- *The application of neuro-imaging technologies has turned the 'gaze' of the clinician from a literal to a simulated reading of the functioning of the human brain.*
- *Localisation is a key organising principle for cognitive neuroscience; it assumes a hard-wired connection of neurons, assigning mental processes to specific regions of the brain.*
- *The process of 'black-boxing' is when scientific and technical work is made invisible by its own successes—Latour.*
- *Cognitive neuroscience presents itself as being able to settle the uncertainty of psychiatric diagnosis by identifying the underlying neural processes of mental illness.*
- *An over-reliance on neuro-imaging has been found to produce a discourse of 'ambivalence' among psychiatrists managing patients with autism spectrum disorder.*

Bibliography

American Psychiatric Association. (2013). *DSM-V: Diagnostic and Statistical Manual of Mental Disorder*. Washington, DC: APA.

Assaf, Y. (2018). New Dimensions for Brain Mapping. *Science, 362*(6418), 994–995.

Bertorelli, T. (2016). Hope and Doubt in the Promise of Neuroimaging: The Case of Autism Spectrum Disorder. *Health, 20*(5), 505–522.

Bleakley, A., & Bligh, J. (2009). Who Can Resist Foucault? *Journal of Medicine and Philosophy, 34*, 368–383.

Cohn, S. (2012). Disrupting Images: Neuroscientific Representations in the Lives in Psychiatric Patients. In S. Choudhury & J. Slaby (Eds.), *Critical Neuroscience: A Handbook of Social and Cultural Contexts of Neuroscience* (pp. 179–194). Chichester: Wiley Blackwell.

Cooper, R., & Shallice, T. (2010). Cognitive Neuroscience: The Troubled Marriage of Cognitive Science and Neuroscience. *Topics in Cognitive Science, 2*, 398–406.

Coopmans, C., Vertesi, J., Lynch, M., & Woolgar, S. (2014). Introduction. In C. Coopmans, J. Vertesi, M. Lynch, & S. Woolgar (Eds.), *Representation in Scientific Practice Revisited* (pp. 1–12). Cambridge, MA: MIT Press.

Cousins, M., & Hussain, A. (1984). *Michel Foucault*. Basingstoke: Macmillan.

Deschauer, M. (2011). Black Box Brain: Anthropological Research on Neurosciences. In P. Gibas, K. Pauknerová, & M. Stella (Eds.), *Non-humans in Social Science: Animals, Spaces, Things*. Cˇervený Kostelec, Czech Rep. Pavel Mervart.

De Rijcke, S., & Beaulieu, A. (2014). Networked Neuroscience: Brain Scans and Visual Knowing at the Intersection of Atlases and Databases. In C. Coopmans, J. Vertesi, M. Lynch, & S. Woolgar (Eds.), *Representation in Scientific Practice Revisited* (pp. 131–152). Cambridge, MA: MIT Press.

Dumit, J. (2014). How (Not) to Do Things with Brain Images. In C. Coopmans, J. Vertesi, M. Lynch, & S. Woolgar (Eds.), *Representation in Scientific Practice Revisited* (pp. 291–313). Cambridge, MA: MIT Press.

Dyer, C. (2010). *Lancet* Retracts Wakefield's MMR Paper. *British Medical Journal, 340*, c396.

Fitzgerald, D. (2014). The Trouble with Brain Imaging: Hope, Uncertainty and Ambivalence in the Neuroscience of Autism. *BioSocieties, 9*(3), 241–261.

Foucault, M. (1967/1989). *Madness and Civilisation*. London: Routledge.

Foucault, M. (1973). *The Birth of the Clinic: An Archaeology of Medical Perception*. London: Tavistock Publications.

Gardner, J., Samuel, G., & Williams, C. (2015). Sociology of Low Expectations: Recalibration as Innovation Work in Biomedicine. *Science, Technology, & Human Values, 40*(6), 998–1021.

Greenfield, A. (2017). *Radical Technologies: The Design of Everyday Life*. London: Verso.

Harrison, B., & Pentalis, C. (2010). Cognitive Subtraction. In I. Stolerman (Ed.), *Encyclopaedia of Psychopharmacology*. Berlin: Springer.

Jay, V. (2000). The Legacy of Jean-Martin Charcot. *Archives of Pathology & Laboratory Medicine, 124*(1), 10–11.

Kessler, R., Bergland, P., & Demler, O. (2005). Lifetime Prevalence and Age-of-Onset Distributions of DSM-IV Disorders in the National Comorbidity Survey Replication. *Archives of General Psychiatry, 62*(6), 593–602.

Latour, B. (1987). *Science in Action: How to Follow Scientists and Engineers through Society*. Cambridge, MA: Harvard University Press.

Latour, B. (1999). *Pandora's Hope: Essays on the Reality of Science Studies*. Cambridge, MA: Harvard University Press.

Legrenzi, P., & Umiltà, C. (2011). *Neuromania: On the Limits of Brain Science*. Oxford: Oxford University Press.

Miller, G. (2003). The Cognitive Revolution: A Historical Perspective. *Trends in Cognitive Science, 7*(3) 141–144.

NHS. (2017). Retrieved May 2019, from www.nhs.uk/news/neurology/could-brain-scans-be-used-to-screen-for-autism/.

Pickersgill, M. (2013). The Social Life of the Brain: Neuroscience in Society. *Current Sociology, 61*(3), 322–340.

Rippon, G. (2019). *The Gendered Brain*. London: The Bodley Head.

Rose, S. (1986). *Molecules and Minds: Essays on Biology and the Social Order*. Buckingham: Open University Press.

Rose, N., & Abi-Rached, J. (2013). *Neuro: The New Brain Sciences and the Management of the Mind*. Princeton, NJ: Princeton University Press.

Tsuji, S. (2013). The Neurogenomics View of Neurological Diseases. *JAMA Neurology, 70*(6), 689–694.

The Neuro-Enculturation of the Social World

5

Abstract

This chapter takes as its starting point the emergence over the past decades of a wide array of 'neuro-disciplines', seeking to identify the neural basis of a whole range of social and economic behaviours and processes of human development. A realist analysis is adopted that acknowledges the scientific basis of neuroscience research into human behaviour but critically assesses the ways in which that research has then been translated and used for commercial, social, and political ends. Four examples of these processes of 'neuro-enculturation' are examined: neurolaw, neuroeconomics, early child development, and cognitive enhancement.

Introduction

At the beginning of the third decade of the twenty-first century, a global infrastructure for neuroscience research is now firmly established, and its research findings are given prominence and promoted within the news media and increasingly inform governmental social and economic policy initiatives. Neuroscience research has now a cultural presence, featuring as plot lines in numerous films, books, and TV series and in gaming and entertainment platforms. Brightly coloured media-friendly brain images derived from fMRI technologies have now entered the popular consciousness, appearing to make the neurosciences accessible to all.

In Chap. 4, the discussion focused on how, for most of the twentieth century, the study of human behaviour was indicated by the prefix *psy-*, linked to a body of psychological research and knowledge. While today, the prefix *neuro-* is invoked in the much the same authoritative manner. But mental disorders are not the only field where brain research is now being applied. An ever-expanding catalogue of 'neuro-disciplines' have emerged in the twenty-first century, pressed into service to identify a neural basis for a whole range of social and economic behaviours, as well as

I. Crinson, *The Biomedical Sciences in Society*,
https://doi.org/10.1007/978-981-15-9523-3_5

processes of human development and enhancement. Four examples will be discussed in this chapter. The phenomenon that is described in this chapter as 'neuro-enculturation' is one that closely identifies the individual self and social processes of behaviour with the activities of our brains. This is an understanding that is increasingly influential in many aspects of social life.

This chapter is both thematically and epistemologically distinct from Chap. 4, which took as its theme the social construction of the neuroscience 'gaze' and the ontological challenges that neuroscience brings to psychiatric constructions of the disordered mind. The focus here is with developing a realist social analysis that acknowledges the scientific legitimacy and contribution of neuroscience research into an understanding of social behaviour, but challenges the attempt to supplant the social scientific analysis of all aspects of human interaction with a biologised brain-based one.

The 'Seductive Allure' of the Neuroscience of Human Behaviour

'Sex, Lies, and Brain Scans: How fMRI reveals what really goes on in our minds' was the title of the winner of the 2017 British Psychological Society Book Award for Popular Science. To quote from the Preface to the book; 'The recent explosion of neuroscience techniques has been game-changing in terms of understanding the healthy brain, and in the development of neuropsychiatric treatments… (T)hrough fMRI, we are beginning to build a deeper understanding of our thoughts, motivations, and behaviours' (Sahakian and Gottwald 2017). The book chapters are variously entitled: 'Can neuroscientists read your mind?'; 'The racial bias hiding in your mind'; 'How moral is your brain'; and 'Show me your brain and I know what you buy'. This book is not written by hack journalists, its authors are an eminent neuropsychologist and a neuroscience PhD student, and the publisher is the Oxford University Press. One of the authors is a former winner of an award for communicating science to the public, which may or may not explain the sensationalist title. The material within the book is rather more circumspect than the title and chapter headings might imply, but nevertheless it offers a largely uncritical account of future applications for fMRI research in understanding human behaviour. *'Sex, Lies, and Brain Scans'* is just one example of a whole raft of popular science publications that look to the neurosciences rather than to the social and economic sciences, or indeed philosophy, to provide explanations for, and a potential resolution of, the iniquities and uncertainties associated with human development and social behaviour. This publishing and media phenomenon can be conceived of as one manifestation of a social process that in this chapter will be termed 'neuro-enculturation'.

Whether these popular science texts (sometimes connected with a spin-off television series) have succeeded in bringing about a transformation in our understanding of human behaviour and subjectivity is a moot point. But this popularisation of neuroscience (generally not including the caveats and limitations frequently included in the original peer-reviewed research paper) has contributed to a wider public interest in the disorders of human cognition and intellectual development.

This burgeoning cultural development is often referred to as 'neuroscientism'. Tom Sorell in his eponymous book describes scientism as; 'a matter of putting too high a value on natural science in comparison with other branches of learning or culture' (1991: 2). The expression neuroscientism is an extension of the notion of 'scientism' in the context of the application of neuroscience research to subjects traditionally outside the domain of the brain sciences. If science is an activity that explores the natural world using rational, replicable, and tested methods, then 'scientism' is its opposite: 'a speculative worldview about the ultimate reality of the universe and its meaning (which) focuses an inordinate amount of its attention on human behaviour and beliefs. Rather than working within carefully constructed boundaries and methodologies established by researchers, it broadly generalizes entire fields of academic expertise and dismisses many of them as inferior' (Burnett 2014). Neuroscientism leads on to a collapsing of biological and cultural distinctions one into the other (Sampson 2017). Jessica Pykett has described the social phenomenon of biological brain-based explanations ('because we are made like that') of complex human processes as 'Brain culture'. She utilises this concept as a short-hand, 'for the circulation, within specific socio-spatial contexts, of a particular approach to human identity, sociality, decision-making, will-power, reasoning and responsibility, which is shaping how citizens govern themselves and how they are governed by others' (Pykett 2017: 29).

The neuroscientists, Legrenzi and Umiltà in their book 'Neuromania', draw attention to what they see as being a particular predilection of the public for 'neuro-explanations'. Citing research carried out at Yale University, they argue that the public is said to be more convinced of some explanation of a social event or phenomenon if it includes a reference to neuroscience; that it gives it 'added value' whether or not that information is correct or not (2011: 61). Raymond Tallis, the philosopher, cultural critic, and clinical scientist, is being highly ironic when he states that, 'the path to a better understanding of our experiences, our motives, our motivations, and, indeed, our very selves, lies through ever more precise ways of observing the brain activity of conscious individuals' (Tallis 2008: 19). In seeking to explain why neuro-imaging research, that draws on a technically sophisticated methodology that few non-specialists can fully understand let alone critique has become so dominant in the popular imagination, Legrenzi and Umiltà (2011: 70) cite the Gestalt principle (see Glossary) of 'multi-stability'. Multi-stability theory is concerned with how we cognitively process complex and what might seem to be contradictory information. The principle asserts that when we perceive something, we "fix" it in our minds and see only that item. Then if we subsequently see it as something else, that new image gets fixed. When we know that something could be one thing or another, it is difficult for us to see both at the same time. As such, '(O)ur perception "flips" between one "stable" image and the other…we don't like uncertainty and like to be consistent, so that when there are two or more ways of seeing something, one perception may become dominant. This dominant perception then occurs first every time we encounter the phenomenon, and so we find it harder to flip to an alternative view' (Straker 2010). The allure of neuroscience fMRI research for non-specialists is therefore seen to reside in the apparently powerful imaging evidence it provides for the location and specificity of cognitive processes and behaviours within identifiable neural pathways. This is a perception that is all too easily becomes 'fixed', rejecting more complex and uncertain explanations for human behaviour. Without delving any deeper into the psychological processes of perception, it is apparent that explanations able to make a simple and direct one-to-one link between a cognitive state and the 'lighting-up' or activation of a particular part of the brain hold a seductive allure for the vast majority of the population who are non-specialists.

Neuroscientific explanations of human behaviour appear to provide an objectively neutral evidence base for policy interventions. Yet, as we shall see, in practice neuroscience research is frequently over-simplified and deployed to support traditional social and moral explanations. This process of translation has been described as 'myth making', the effect of which has been to 'strip away moral debate and delimit the number of policy and professional responses' to the human cost of deep-seated social and economic problems (Wastell and White 2017: 90). Broer and Pickersgill's (2015) documentary analysis has examined the ways in which neuroscience findings and concepts have come to 'find their way' into official UK health and social and policy reports. Their conclusions point to neuroscience being used to both support and give authority to what are essentially politicised definitions of personal and parental responsibility for early years child development. Neuroscience research has also been used to provide a scientific basis for the problematising of adolescence as a period of social and physical development. The irony of the use of neuroscience research in policy statements to ascribe specific social problems to the functioning of brains is that: '(T)he solution that they plea for is often a relational one, where parents have a more loving relationship with their children and understand their teenagers better, and where people care for and understand the behaviour of those with dementia' (Broer and Pickersgill 2015: 60).

▶ **Theory Box 5.1 A Critical Realist Reading of Neuroscience as Applied to Social Behaviour** Critical realism (CR) is a philosophical framework of analysis that emphasises the importance of giving attention to both the ontological as well as the epistemological claims of science. It recognises the existence of a stratified world, but with each strata of reality having its own set of non-reducible properties and mechanisms understood in terms of new or 'emergent powers' (discussed in Chap. 2).

It is on this basis that CR would not seek to deny the relevance of a neuropsychological contribution to the reading of social behaviour. This is because there is clearly a biological basis for the material existence of human beings, in cells, brains, and bodies. But CR would seek to emphasise the importance of a socially situated emergence in contextualising human behaviour, thoughts, feelings, and reflections. Humans, 'do not simply "behave", they also conduct themselves in moral orders that they contribute to, are mindful of and many times try to change' (Pilgrim 2019: 148). A CR analysis would acknowledge, but seek to go beyond, the constructionist framing of neuropsychological approaches as reductionist. The CR critique is that neuroscience will always hold the presumption that higher level social phenomena such as behaviour is ontologically indistinct from lower level phenomena, such as neurochemical activity or neuroanatomical structures.

In pointing to the uniqueness with human 'being', CR would recognise an asymmetrical relationship existing between the biophysical realm and the social realm. The principle of emergence at different levels of reality points to higher level phenomena such as social processes and structures possessing properties that are independent of, and cannot be predicted by the lower levels of chemistry and biology. So that while human neurobiology plays a contributory role in any given psychological process, 'once these higher level phenomena emerge in distinct forms, they exert a recursive influence upon the operation of the lower level mechanisms that give rise to them, acting as constraints' (Healey and Hodgkinson 2014: 773).

So while human perceptions, goals, and needs are cognitive states that arise from neural activity in certain parts of the brain, once established these higher level mental events then serve to *mediate* the operation of those same neural stimuli. There is therefore an important ontological difference between the assumption that higher level functions of cognition applied to socially-situated human activities make use of lower level neurological processes, and assuming that these same processes determine the behaviour of that individual and the wider operation of social systems (Healey and Hodgkinson 2014: 774).

For example, neuroscientists are potentially able to identify the neural substrates of impulsive behaviour, pointing to its manifestation as forms of self-interest in experimental work involving economic games ('neuroeconomics'—described in detail below). But this neurocentric approach ignores the role played by higher level social rules, both formal and informal, established through processes of socialisation, group norms, and organisational culture, in constraining impulsive behaviours. A socially situated CR perspective points to the ways in which social neuroscience 'would benefit from focusing on how organizations influence the neural substrates of motivation and emotion that are generative mechanisms of impulsiveness' (Healey and Hodgkinson 2014: 781).

Neuro-enculturation 1: Neurolaw

Neurolaw is a rapidly developing field of interdisciplinary research that seeks to apply the methodology of the neurosciences to matters of jurisprudence, and in particular criminal law. Criminal and civil law has since early modern times looked to the human mind and mental states as a basis for understanding criminal behaviour and individual responsibility. Over the last hundred years and more, legal systems have recognised the pertinence of cognitive deficits and psychological diagnoses as a form of legal defence. Neuroscience reprsesents a tantalising next step in the involvement of science in determining the balance of individual guilt and punishment.

A recent editorial in the *Journal of Psychiatry and Neuroscience* identified three areas of potential application for neuroscience research within legal systems: revision, assessment, and intervention (Meynan 2016). 'Revision' refers to whether neuroscience research findings should lead onto revisions of the law and legal practices. An extreme and notorious example would be the claim that neuroscience is able to demonstrate that 'free will', a key principle of moral philosophy that underpins the majority of existing criminal justice systems, is an illusion and cannot constitute a scientific basis for determining guilt and punishment. Given that the notion of free will is the basis for determining criminal responsibility, a rejection of its legal viability would logically require a major revision of criminal law in terms of guilt and retribution. If free will does not exit, then there can be no defence plea of mental insanity. The insanity defence being a legal concept not a clinical one. To successfully use this defence, a defendant must demonstrate that at the time a crime was committed, they were suffering from a severe mental illness. As such, they would be incapable of differentiating right from wrong, so unable to understand the nature of their crime, and cannot therefore be held legally accountable. If the insanity plea becomes meaningless because of neuroscience evidence, then psychiatric evaluations of defendants would also become obsolete. The second area identified for the application of neuroscience is in the 'assessment' of defendants, witnesses, and prospective jurors. Lawyers may in future be able to pose questions such as, what is the risk of recidivism for this particular defendant? What does the witness remember exactly, and are they lying in their evidence? Is this prospective juror biased against certain groups of people? And such questions may be answered with the help of neuroscience. The third area of neuroscience application concerns potential interventions. This might in future include neuro-based treatment options that reduce the risk of recidivism (Meynan 2016: 3–4).

One practical example of the involvement of neuroscience in the legal system is the process of attempting to scientifically determine the legal age for criminal responsibility. Currently, the legal systems in the majority of countries now have some form of age-based limits or parameters for determining individual responsibility, that is, only over-18s can vote and legally drink alcohol, and so on. That these age limits are linked to cultural conceptions of adolescent maturity is evidenced in the wide differences to be found in the minimum age that children can be arrested and charged with a crime in legal systems across the world. Even within the

European Union, differences in the legal age of criminal responsibility are quite marked. The UK criminalises children at a lower age than any other EU country; this is set at 10 years of age where it has been since the 1963 (when it changed from 8 years of age!). In Germany, it is currently at age 14, in Sweden it is 15, while in Portugal it is 16. The social and cultural conventions that underpin these legal assumptions of adolescent maturity and immaturity are qualitatively different from that of any neuroscience-based approach. Neuro-psychology would generally conceptualise adolescence as a developmental period marked by brain immaturity and by higher levels of risk-taking.

On this basis, Dumit (2014) has posed the question of whether neuroscience is able to draw a 'bright line' that can demonstrate the parameters of responsibility that can be expected of the adolescent brain, and so scientifically address the problem of what to do with adolescents who break the law? He answers his rhetorical question by asserting that neuroscience 'should not and cannot be a neutral arbiter of efforts to assign classes of people to either immaturity or dangerousness, because they are embedded within the very categories they are being asked to resolve' (2014: 293). That is, when neuro-imaging research attempts to identify markers or evidence of immaturity, it becomes difficult to disentangle the biological from the social assumptions of what constitutes maturity-immaturity. The point being that analytical dangers arise when reifying cognitive maturity on the basis of categories that have their origins in social constructions. Dumit goes on to make the point that at present there are no agreed neuroscientific criteria that can replace judicial determinations of maturity or decision-making capacity. If neuroscientific findings are used in court they are almost only used to reinforce stereotypes of adolescent riskiness (Dumit 2014: 307).

Neural connections in the brain change throughout life not just in adolescence, so that any notion of biological maturity as a 'realised state' is a misleading one. In future, there may well be neuroscientific measures of adolescence that would call into question the precise association of immaturity with age. It then might be discovered that some middle age men are immature by this measure and some teenagers are mature, regardless of their actual behaviour, criminal or otherwise. This would then demonstrate 'the conundrum that the neurosciences are in when they address social categories of persons and attempt to put forward scientific claims about a category' (Dumit 2014: 296).

Neuro-enculturation 2: Neuroeconomics

While there are clear connections between mainstream cognitive neuroscience and neuroeconomics, the latter's focus on the neural basis of decision-making has largely proceeded on a separate path (Winecoff and Huettel 2017: 408–409). This interdisciplinary field has been concerned to link the disciplines of economics, psychology, and neuroscience in order to develop analytical tools to better understand and intervene to effect change in the processes of economic decision-making. Its modus operandi is to pose a series of rhetorical questions such as: 'How do uncertainty and risk shape decisions? How are others' rewards and risks incorporated into social decisions? What changes the objective qualities of a reward into subjective utility for an individual? If these questions of causality can be addressed with intellectual vigour and robustness, then the economic rewards are potentially huge. This may well explain why many of the leading universities around the world have set-up laboratories or centres for neuroeconomics. Research papers explicitly presented under the banner of neuroeconomics now frequently appear in the leading journals of science journals such as *Nature* and *Science*.

Historically, the cognitive and neuronal processes that may (or may not) influence individual choice were never part of mainstream economic theory. However, as an applied academic discipline, economics has for many decades been concerned with the factors that shape individual decision-making. The first attempts at developing an explanation are generally said to have begun in the late 1940s with 'game theory', a mathematical approach to understanding rational strategic decision-making. At best, game theory was a form of thought experiment concerned with an ideal-type world where all the information needed to make rational choices was readily available. The assumptions underpinning this mathematical approach never had any basis in the real world. Game theory had been jettisoned by the early 1970s in favour of psychological theories of judgement, an approach that sought to assess the perception and handling of information in circumstances of uncertainty; this became known as 'utility theory'. Underpinning this research was an attempt to statistically model rational choice for the purposes of inferring the probabilistic courses of action available to individuals in financial commodity markets. However, overtime the limitations of the view that an individual's actions are determined by their desired goal, and their choice of how best way to reach that goal became apparent. From experimental work, it was demonstrated that in the real world, individuals don't always make logical economic choices. This understanding then led onto the development at the end of the twentieth century of what become known as 'behavioural economics'. This field starts from an entirely different premise to that of traditional economics. It assumes that humans utilise cognitive shortcuts when making purchasing or investment decisions that are subject to all sorts unconscious personal and cultural biases, which in turn makes them vulnerable to a range of pre-existing and subtle influences (Pykett 2016: 81–82).

Fulsomely reviewed and widely available, the core tenets of behavioural economics began to exert an influence on the strategies of governments that were aimed at bringing about change in those attitudes and behaviours seen as being problematic to the health and welfare of their citizens. This range of initiatives subsequently became known as 'nudge' policies, the term deriving from Thaler and Sunstein's eponymous popular science book published in 2008. Such policies targeted behaviour change linked to positive reinforcement and reward incentives. Examples of such initiatives to persuade citizens 'to make better choices for themselves' in the UK, Australia, and USA, include anti-smoking, anti-obesity, recycling, and the take-up of personal pension schemes with the goal of reducing the pensions 'burden' on the state. These initiatives were designed to gain the compliance of the public without coercion or the formal regulation of 'undesirable' or 'ill-considered' behaviour. Critics, however, have argued that such 'nudges' can be misused and in essence constitute a form of social engineering.

The goal of neuroeconomics is to build a neuroscience-based unified model of human choice. Research has focused on the neural activity involved when individuals make economic decisions, thereby generating a physiological-based model for the known inconsistencies in the rational choice model of neoclassical economics. Studies have sought to integrate fMRI imaging data with single-neuron measurements in non-human primates, in order to identify statistically significant correlations between decisions and localised changes in brain blood flow and blood oxygenation, coupled to underlying neuronal activity in areas such as the ventral striatum (VS) and the ventromedial prefrontal cortex (VMPFC). Building on such findings, neuroeconomists have contended that these localised areas of the brain constitute the core of a neural system for value-based learning and decision-making (Fumagalli 2015: 89). But there are both empirical and conceptual reasons to question the assertion that stimulated neuronal activity is the key determinant of behaviour. It is one thing to identify short-term stimulus-response rewards producing behavioural responses in non-human primates within the artificial pared-down environment of the laboratory, but quite another when it comes to predicting the long-term non-stimulus-bound investment and purchasing choices made by individuals that is the focus of economists (Fumagalli 2015: 90).

The underlying assumption of neuroeconomic research is that there are a limited and therefore potentially identifiable set of neurobiological and neurochemical processes that result in decision-making and behaviour. This is essentially a form of monism, the philosophical view that there are a unified set of laws underlying all of nature, as opposed to pluralist doctrines that see many kinds of things at work in nature. Monism in neuroscience leads implicitly to the position that cognitive abilities are ascribed to the brain rather than the individual. This understanding has been described as a 'mereological fallacy'. The assumption that properties such as learning and understanding should be ascribed to the brain, or even a small substrate of the brain, rather than to the whole behaving person (Smit and Hacker 2014—cited in Krakauer et al. 2017. 483). There are many neuroscientists and economists who would question the sustainability of the claim that categories drawn from the biological world can explain the processes of decision-making and economic behaviour in a multi-layered and complex social world. As John Krakauer and his neuroscience colleagues have noted; '(T)oo often in neuroscience causal efficacy is taken as equal to understanding' (2017: 483). Many orthodox economists are sceptical of the claims of what they term BES ('behavioural economics in the scanner'), this being the view that neuroeconomics is too dependent on the use of fMRI data, seen as at best first-order observations rather than worked through deductive science (Harrison and Ross 2012: 88). Neuroeconomics would therefore appear to have a rather large blind spot, and this would be the social and cultural context of individual decision-making and economic choice in an 'imperfect market' (see Glossary).

Knowledge of neural activity and connections is not synonymous with knowing exactly what these neural structures are doing to cause behaviour. An analogy would be that understanding the game of chess is not dependent on knowing anything about the material out of which the pieces and board are made (Krakauer et al. 2017: 483). In addressing the question of whether the neuronal causal-mechanistic explanations of decision-making found in neuroeconomics are sufficient and necessary to explain economic behaviour, Krakauer et al. (2017) argue that first we have to ask why is the brain performing this behaviour, and only then ask how is it doing it. To address these questions then requires the application of higher level philosophy of science concepts that are able to point to effects that go beyond the biological boundaries of neural pathways. Only then can the components of a neural mechanism be seen as doing different things when the mechanism as a whole operates or behaves when it is embedded in a multi-variable environment (Krakauer et al. 2017: 485). We learn little when we study mechanisms in isolation and at a reductionist level, for this does not take account of the emergence that follows interactivity in a complex environment. These are conclusions that reflect, if not explicitly, then certainly implicitly, the 'depth reality' characteristic of the natural world; an understanding consistent with a CR methodology (see Theory Box 5.1 above).

Finally, while 'nudge' programmes of behaviour change may be described as paternalistic, they are relatively equitable by comparison with the potential of interventionist policies based on the monistic assumptions of neuroeconomics. The latter would effectively identify and place individuals, 'along a spectrum of competency in relation to their tendency toward short-termist and potentially self-defeating behaviours…such policies would be by their very nature be highly interventionist for those citizens marked out as more irrational or impulsive' (Pykett 2016: 88). A potentially real world actualisation of the 'previsualised' thought crimes dramtically portrayed in the 'Minority Report' movie. The practical implications of constructing interventions based on the biologistic assumptions of neuroeconomics would be challenging indeed for the ethical and moral principles underpinning democratic political systems.

Neuro-enculturation 3: Early Years Development

The earliest manifestation of the national state intervening in the relationship between a child and their parents in the UK was over 130 years ago. Known as the 1899 'children's charter', this was one of the first examples of child welfare legislation designed to protect children from cruelty and exploitation by their own parents (legislation to 'protect' children in factory employment having occurred sixty years earlier). By the end of the nineteenth century, the scope of Victorian Age public health that had focused on improving sanitation and the prevention of disease in the rapidly expanding cities had broadened out to encompass middle-class concerns about the social and moral welfare of children of working-class families. Over the course of the twentieth century, a foundational position developed within the emergent field of child development psychology or 'developmental psychology', which was the notion that the first two or three years predetermined the rest of a child's life. These psychological theories were firmly established several decades before the advent of neuroscience research in this field. Yet they were built upon the conviction that 'every experience produces a permanent change somewhere in the central nervous system and therefore the earliest experiences provide the scaffolding for the child's future thought and behaviour' (Kagan 1998: 86; cited in Wastell and White 2017: 10).

Over the course of the second half of the twentieth century, it was these research assumptions of developmental psychology that came to both define and proscribe 'normal' child development. Childhood became something that was seen to be divided-up into a series of sequential biological stages or 'milestones' through which a child had to successfully pass. The notion of 'childrearing' associated with what had hitherto been seen as an autonomous and largely instinctive role played by mothers and fathers gradually came to be replaced with the designation 'parenting'. By the 1970s, such developmental psychological theories were being popularised in authoritative 'guides' to parenting. The sociological concept that attempts to capture this changing cultural and political environment in which child psychologists were granted the legitimacy to guide parents in how best to raise and nurture their children is termed 'parental-determinism'. This is a cultural process that has in more recent years largely re-shaped the self-expectations and responsibilities of parents in raising their own children. Attention was now focused on the parent-child relation, often rendered as potentially problematic by child development specialists, and in need of their expertise to avoid 'deficiencies' in a child's cognitive development. By scrutinising the minutiae of interactions, smiling, eye contact, and so forth, the new profession of child development specialist was charged with spotting those at risk of developing social and emotional maladjustment: 'And when risk was spotted, it must be pre-empted' (Wastell and White 2017: 12). Drawing on Bowlby's (1973) highly influential attachment theory, parenting had by the end of the twentieth century become 'repositioned as both a potential cause and solution to the "problem" of the developing child, and the quality of parenting rather than the child itself, come to be a major focus of state policy' (Lowe et al. 2015: 205).

Some two decades ago, a neuroscience-based approach began to assert itself within most areas of psychology (as discussed in Chap. 4), and the field of child development was no exception. Neuroscience research was used to construct a portrayal of the first three years of life as a period of particular neural vulnerability and as offering the potential for new forms of intervention. In the context of early childhood development, this approach drew on the emerging neuroplastic understanding that the brain is not hard-wired for life at birth, but that a child's environment can serve to enhance motor and cognitive functions, or interfere with normal behavioural development. Although there are not many studies of pathological plasticity in the developing brain, what examples there are usually include foetal alcohol spectrum disorder and the effects of severe prenatal stress, both of which have been shown to markedly reduce the complexity of neurons in the prefrontal cortex (Kolb and Gibb 2011: 268). Other neuroscience-based research suggests that exposure to 'harsh and unpredictable childhood conditions (e.g., parental neglect) is associated with greater volume and reactivity of the amygdala, a portion of the brain that is responsible for vigilance and emotional responsiveness to threat' (Simons and Klopack 2015: 576). It should be noted that all these findings are largely based on the outcomes of experimental studies involving rats and their offspring and various manipulations of their environment. For clear ethical reasons, research with children in the far more complex social world in which humans interact and build relationships over time is not possible.

Despite the many complexities and uncertainties that characterise the application of neuro-imaging research, particularly in the context of the cognitive development of young infants, policy-makers and opinion-formers have not held back from attempting to translate the neuroscience to support social and welfare policy initiatives. Wastell and White (2017) have identified three core assumptions about the findings of the neuroscience of early years which are then incorporated into the development of social and educational policy. Firstly, the assumption that the first three years of life represent a period of 'biological exuberance' in the development of brain connectivity, characterised by an explosive growth in the number of synapses. Secondly, that this constitutes a once-and-for-all 'critical period'. Third, that an enriched and stimulating environment will augment brain development, 'boosting brain power' (Wastell and White 2017: 97). In 2001, the government incorporated the recommendations of a report entitled 'Birth to Three Matters' into the design of its national Sure Start programme. Sure Start was targeted at parents and children under the age of four living in the most disadvantaged areas, with the goal of delivering a coordinated service to assist parents in supporting their children's learning skills, health and well-being, and social and emotional development. The literature review accompanying the report contained nearly one hundred references to brain development research. It extensively cites both US and UK research in order to emphasise the ways in which early childhood experiences affect: '(T)he "design" of the brain, and influence the nature and extent of adult capabilities…impact on the way the brain is "wired" as well as creating the context for development and learning…(*whilst recognising that*) brain development is non-linear: at certain times there are "sensitive" periods at which conditions for particular kinds of learning are optimal' (David et al. 2003: 123).

Over time this more neuro-deterministic approach to child development began to appear regularly in official policy. For example, in the 2006 Cabinet Office report entitled *Reaching Out: An Action Plan on Social Exclusion*, the following statement can be found: 'The child who is spoken to will develop speech and language neural systems, and the child who has motor practice and exploration opportunities will develop neural systems which allow walking, running and fine motor control. The child who is nurtured and loved will develop the neural networks which mediate empathy, compassion and the capacity to form health relationships' (Cabinet Office 2006—cited in Lowe et al. 2015: 203). This understanding has subsequently been incorporated into interventions aimed at maximising cognitive development in the 'time sensitive' early years in the UK. The conclusions of a more recent Department of Education publication entitled an *Impact Study on Early Education Use and Child Outcomes up to Age Three* (Melhuish et al. 2017) are based almost exclusively on evidence from neuroscience and psychological research to demonstrate that variations in early years cognitive and socio-emotional developmental outcomes are almost exclusively associated with home environment. It is on this basis that the report recommends that 'disadvantaged groups may be considered to have more to gain from early childhood education and care (Melhuish et al. 2017: 71–72).

Outside of formal social and welfare interventions, parents of young children are encouraged to become active consumers of 'neurobiological discourses that present the brains of babies, children and young adults as plastic objects to be cared for, but also as biological constants that are determinative of behavior and subjectivity' (Pickersgill 2013: 329). These are the discourses to be found in an exponentially increasing number of 'self-help' books, web-based blogs, and chat rooms aimed at new parents and offering neurological-based advice on stimulating child development. This is a form of 'parental determinism' for the twenty-first century, one that positions parents as both the cause and solution to the 'problem' of the developing child. Neuroscience has arguably been deployed to shift the source of educational underachievement and psychological distress as an outcome of social and economic inequality to that of problematic and individualised parental behaviour.

Neuro-enculturation 4: Cognitive Enhancement

If neuroscience research is increasingly defining normative human behaviour, it is also being drawn upon to find 'solutions' to overcome these 'deficits' in performance. One such area is the claims being made for the enhancement of cognitive functioning through the use (or misuse) of prescription pharmaceuticals such as methylphenidate, (dextro-) amphetamine, donepezil, and modafinil. These drugs are prescribed for a variety of disorders, including attention-deficit hyperactivity disorder (ADHD), postural orthostatic tachycardia syndrome, Alzheimer's disease or dementia, shift work sleep disorder, and narcolepsy (Müller and Schumann 2011). The enhancement claims made for these pharmaceuticals include memory, intelligence, linguistic skills, and the ability to focus on intellectual tasks, as well as a heightening of sense perception. These are enhancements that students studying for exams, and 'burned-out' workers might well value. It is on this basis that some social scientists have argued that this development is 'indicative of a broader societal move away from viewing dependence on pharmaceuticals as a weakness, to instead considering their consumption as desirable or even essential in order to fully participate in society' (Martin et al. 2011).

The drug 'Modafinil' first came to the UK market as a pharmaceutical treatment for narcolepsy in 2002. Its licence has since been extended to cover excessive daytime sleepiness (EDS) and is also prescribed 'off-label' (see Glossary) as a 'wake-promoting' drug to overcome conditions causing fatigue and sleep deprivation. On the basis of these effects modafinil has been cited as a 'performance enhancer'. Here the term 'enhancement' is used to include both therapeutic and non-therapeutic effects, with any attempts to distinguish between the two being seen as arbitrary and not analytically useful (Synofzik 2009—cited in Coveney 2011: 208). In 2012, the European Medicines Agency (EMA) advised that modafinil should be only prescribed for narcolepsy because of its association with psychiatric problems, together with the consequences of its misuse by healthy populations, especially university students. Despite these cautions, it is regularly reported in the media and elsewhere that the illicit use of cognitive enhancers continue to grow, in part because they are seen as to be 'safe' and improve performance.

In a skill-driven and knowledge-based society, it is often claimed that success correlates with one's cognitive abilities, so that any means of 'enhancement' is seen to be a competitive good that can give some people an advantage over others in gaining employment, advancing careers and earning a higher income: '(T)o be "smarter" than other people is considered to be an asset in many situations and it is assumed that those who are not cognitively enhanced could be disadvantaged' (Coveney 2011: 210). To investigate these social assumptions, Coveney (2011) conducted qualitative interviews with two social groups often linked with the use of cognitive enhancement drugs, shift workers, and full-time students. The perception of modafinil held by individuals in both groups was as a 'therapeutic technology'. For shift workers it was seen as a way to repair a deficit in work performance and restore 'normal' levels of cognitive functioning, as a safety tool preventing potential accidents or mistakes. While the student accounts of using modafinil were 'dominated by intrigue and temptation', its role as a study aid was 'readily imagined'. Yet amongst these students, it was also found that there was a general scepticism about the potential of the drug as a cognitive enhancer to improve academic performance; 'sounds too good to be true' said one interviewee. The idea of using a prescription medicine as an aid to study outside of formal medical approval was generally viewed by the student interviewees as an illicit and inappropriate use of a prescription drug. Fellow students who were known to be using the drug were frequently perceived as 'cheats'. The view of both the shift workers and students was that cognitive enhancement drugs should only be used if someone was experiencing 'real problems'. Yet when both these groups were asked to imagine a future scenario in which cognitive enhancement drugs were widely available over the counter, the use of modafinil as a study aid or safety tool was then constructed as a personal, autonomous choice.

A similarly themed research study was conducted with students and staff of four German universities, this time utilising a self-completed questionnaire additional to a randomised control trial (Sattler et al. 2013). The study was predicated on the social psychological utility-based rational choice theory (described in the section on Neuroeconomics above), in which participants were asked to rate their willingness to take a hypothetical cognitive enhancing drug. The drug's effect in increasing mental performance was experimentally varied across the study groups in terms of the likelihood of experiencing increases in mental performance and the probability of experiencing side-effects. The aim of the study was therefore to assess both the staff and student's 'internalised norms' to abstain from cognitive enhancing drug use. Unsurprisingly perhaps, an increase in the perceived utility of the drug to enhance cognitive processes also increased the probability of both groups to use it, and vice versa. This was a process that was seen to 'indicate that users are neither naive nor exclusively benefit oriented' (Sattler et al. 2013). The study looked not only at rational deliberation but also at whether the use of cognitively enhancing drugs would be influenced by internalised social norms. The internalised social norm being assessed was the extent to which using the drug without any medical indication was deemed to be morally dubious or not. Here, the study found that if such moral norms were strongly 'internalised', they significantly reduced the willingness of the participants to use the drug, even if its utility was perceived as high. For the authors, this finding can be explained by the fact that a violation of internalised norms can result in internal penalties such as psychological costs: 'As internalized norms against cognitive enhancing drug use increased, the effect of utility on the decision to take this medication was reduced…(S)trongly internalized norms work as a filter to refrain from using drugs without deliberation' (Sattler et al. 2013).

The findings of Sattler et al.'s (2013) study are valuable in contextualising the neuro-enculturation process. The assumptions of rational choice theory linked to neuropsychological models of decision-making would dictate that the research participants in both of the studies cited would use cognitive enhancing drugs if convinced of their utility in improving memory retention. However, the strength of internalised social norms in both studies was such that there was a general moral condemnation of using drugs to enhancement performance or 'cheat'. Social norms were also seen to underpin the question of illicit use of such drugs without medical authority, that is, prescribed for a recognised condition. The question that then arises is whether cognitive enhancement through the use of drugs will ever be legitimised as a new social norm? One that would represent a rejection of more humanistic and moral precepts of 'doing your best'. At present in the UK, the sanctions on the use of cognitive enhancing drugs appear to rely solely on the beliefs and attitudes of individuals themselves. Government has limited its responsibility to publicising the negative side-effects of such drugs including psychological addiction and negative physiological effects such as fatal arrhythmias.

Concluding Comments

Martin Pickersgill has issued the following exhortation to social scientists concerned to examine the impact of the new fields of neuroscience as they have played out at the social and cultural level: '(W)e must be wary: not only of claims from neuroscientists and other actors about the potentiality of studies of the brain and the innovations they can and should engender, but also of highly theorized social scientific accounts that might over-play the novelty and import of neuroscience' (Pickersgill 2013: 332). The social scientific literature that has been reviewed and assessed within this chapter largely derives from a realist position. This approach acknowledges the existence of reciprocal interactions between neuroscience and social life, while at the same recognising the necessity of developing a critical analysis of, 'the ways in which neuroscience increasingly functions as a screen upon which to project everyday values about mental life, personhood, and kinds of people' (Slaby and Choudhury 2012: 7).

Chapter Summary—Key Points

- *For most of the twentieth century, the scientific study of human behaviour was primarily indicated by the prefix 'psy-', today that prefix is primarily 'neuro-'.*
- *Neuroscientism is a key element of this process of neuro-enculturation, a collapsing of biological and cultural distinctions one into the other.*
- *Neuroscience represents a tantalising next step in the involvement of science in determining the balance of individual guilt and punishment in criminal law.*
- *The goal of neuroeconomics is to provide a neuronal-based unified theory of human choice and economic decision-making.*
- *The practical implications of constructing interventions based on the assumptions of neuroeconomics would be challenging for democratic ethical and moral principles.*
- *In the twentieth century it was the research assumptions of developmental psychology that came to both define and proscribe 'normal' child development.*
- *In the twenty-first century, neuroscience research is being used to construct a portrayal of the first three years of life as a period of particular neural vulnerability.*
- *The early development findings are largely based on experimental studies involving rats and their offspring and various manipulations of their environment.*
- *Neurobiology presents the brains of babies and children as plastic objects to be cared for, but also as biological constants that are determinative of behaviour and subjectivity.*
- *In a knowledge-based society, it is often claimed that success correlates with one's cognitive abilities, so that any means of 'enhancement' is seen to be a competitive good.*
- *Will the use of cognitive enhancing drugs becomes the new norm, or will this biologising of human behaviour be challenged by our humanistic and moral precepts?*

Bibliography

Bowlby, J. (1973). *Separation: Anger and Anxiety (Volume 2—Attachment and Loss)*. New York: Basic Books.

Broer, T., & Pickersgill, M. (2015). Targeting Brains, Producing Responsibilities: The Use of Neuroscience within British Social Policy. *Social Science and Medicine, 132*, 54–61.

Burnett, T. (2014) *What Is Scientism*? American Association for the Advancement of Science—Dialogue Science Ethics. Retrieved September 2019, from www.aaas.org/programs/dialogue-science-ethics-and-religion/what-scientism.

Cabinet Office. (2006). *Reaching Out: An Action Plan on Social Exclusion*. London: Cabinet Office.

Coveney, C. (2011). Cognitive Enhancement? Exploring Modafinil Use in Social Context. In M. Pickergill & I. Van Keulan (Eds.), *Sociological Reflections on the Neurosciences* (pp. 203–228). Bingley: Emerald.

David, T., Gooch, K., Powell, S., & Abbott, L. (2003). *Birth to Three Matters: A Review of the Literature Compiled to Inform the Framework to Support Children in Their Earliest Years*. Department of Education and Skills—Research Report RR444. London: DfES Publications.

Dumit, J. (2014). How (Not) to Do Things with Brain Images. In C. Coopmans, J. Vertesi, M. Lynch, & S. Woolgar (Eds.), *Representation in Scientific Practice Revisited* (pp. 291–313). Cambridge, MA: MIT Press.

Fumagalli, R. (2015). Five Theses on Neuroeconomics. *Journal of Economic Methodology, 23*(1), 77–96.

Harrison, G., & Ross, D. (2012). The Methodologies of Neuroeconomics. In C. Marchionni & J. Vromen (Eds.), *Neuroeconomics: Hype or Hope?* (pp. 85–96). London: Routledge.

Healey, M., & Hodgkinson, G. (2014). Rethinking the Philosophical and Theoretical Foundations of Organizational Neuroscience: A Critical Realist Alternative. *Human Relations, 67*(7), 765–792.

Kagan, J. (1998). *Three Seductive Ideas*. Harvard, MA: Harvard University Press.

Kolb, B., & Gibb, R. (2011). Brain Plasticity and Behaviour in the Developing Brain. *Journal of the Canadian Academy of Child and Adolescent Psychiatry, 20*(4), 265–276.

Krakauer, J., Ghazanfar, A., Gomez-Marin, A., MacIver, M., & Poeppel, P. (2017). Neuroscience Needs Behavior: Correcting a Reductionist Bias. *Neuron, 93*, 480–490.

Legrenzi, P., & Umiltà, C. (2011). *Neuromania: On the Limits of Brain Science*. Oxford: Oxford University Press.

Lowe, P., Lee, E., & Macvarish, J. (2015). Biologising Parenting: Neuroscience Discourse, English Social and Public Health Policy and Understandings of the Child. *Sociology of Health and Illness, 37*(2), 198–211.

Martin, P., Brown, N., Coveney, C., & Williams, S. (2011). Pharmaceutical Cognitive Enhancement: Interrogating the Ethics, Addressing the Issues. In I. Segev & H. Markham (Eds.), *Augmenting Cognition* (pp. 179–192). Lausanne: EPFL Press.

Melhuish, E., Gardiner, J., & Morris, S. (2017). *Study of Early Education and Development (SEED): Impact Study on Early Education Use and Child Outcomes up to Age Three*. London: DfES Publications.

Meynan, G. (2016). Neurolaw: Recognizing Opportunities and Challenges for Psychiatry. *Journal of Psychiatry and Neuroscience, 41*(1), 3–5.

Müller, C., & Schumann, G. (2011). To Use or Not to Use: Expanding the View on Non-Addictive Psychoactive Drug Consumption and Its Implications. *Behavioral and Brain Sciences, 34*, 328–347.

Pickersgill, M. (2013). The Social Life of the Brain: Neuroscience in Society. *Current Sociology, 61*(3), 322–340.

Pilgrim, D. (2019). Mental Health, Subjectivities and Forms of Neuroscience: A Critical Realist Examination. *Social Theory and Health., 17*, 140–157.

Pykett, J. (2016). From Global Economic Change to Neuromolecular Capitalism. In J. De Vos & E. Pluth (Eds.), *Neuroscience and Critique: Exploring the Limits to the Neurological Turn* (pp. 81–99). London: Routledge.

Pykett, J. (2017). *Brain Culture: Shaping Policy through Neuroscience*. Bristol: Policy Press.

Sahakian, B., & Gottwald, J. (2017). *Sex, Lies, and Brain Scans: How fMRI Reveals What Really Goes on in Our Minds*. Oxford: Oxford University Press.

Sampson, A. (2017). *The Assemblage Brain: Sense Making in Neuroculture*. Minneapolis: University of Minnesota Press.

Sattler, S., Sauer, C., Mehlkop, G., & Graeff, P. (2013). The Rationale for Consuming Cognitive Enhancement Drugs in University Students and Teachers. *PLOS ONE, 8*(7), e68821.

Simons, R., & Klopack, E. (2015). 'The Times They Are A-Changin' Gene Expression, Neuroplasticity, and Developmental Research. *Journal of Youth and Adolescence, 44*, 573–580.

Slaby, J., & Choudhury, S. (2012). Introduction: Critical Neuroscience—Between Lifeworld and Laboratory. In S. Choudhury & J. Slaby (Eds.), *Critical Neuroscience: A Handbook of Social and Cultural Contexts of Neuroscience* (pp. 1–26). Chichester: Wiley Blackwell.

Smit, H., & Hacker, S. (2014). Seven Misconceptions About the Mereological Fallacy: A Compilation for the Perplexed. *Erkenntis, 79*, 1077–1097.
Sorell, T. (1991). *Scientism: Philosophy and the Infatuation with Science*. New York: Routledge.
Straker, D. (2010). Changing Minds. Retrieved July 2019, from http://changingminds.org/.
Synofzik, M. (2009). Ethically Justified, Clinically Applicable Criteria for Physician Decision-Making in Psychopharmacological Enhancement. *Neuroethics, 2*(2), 89–102.
Tallis, R. (2008). The Limitations of a Neurological Approach to Art. *Lancet, 372*, 19–20.
Wastell, D., & White, S. (2017). *Blinded by Science: The Social Implications of Epigenetics and Neuroscience*. Bristol: Policy Press.
Winecoff, A., & Huettel, S. (2017). Cognitive Control and Neuroeconomics. In T. Egner (Ed.), *The Wiley Handbook of Cognitive Control* (pp. 408–421). Chichester: John Wiley & Sons Ltd.

Personalised Medicine in a Post-Genomic Era

6

Abstract

This chapter examines the post-Human Genome Project promissory visions for radically new forms of genomic-based therapeutic interventions. It critically discusses the roles played by Big Pharma, biotechnology companies, and the government in supporting and investing in these visions of the future. The discussion then moves onto a prospective analysis of pharmacogenomics as the key pillar of what is now described as 'personal' or more accurately 'precision medicine'. This is followed by an assessment of the health economics of pharmacogenomics and the social implications of 'personal genomics' associated with the potential of molecular-based diagnostics to enable individuals to manage their health disease susceptibilities and health risks with more certainty.

Introduction

This chapter will assess the current state of applied genomic science twenty years on from the completion of the Human Genome Project. The visions generated by genomic scientists, government, and Big Pharma in the wake of this 'post-genomic revolution' were largely focused on the potential for the development of a new 'personalised' medicine, one linked with molecular-based diagnostics and pharmacogenomic interventions. These developments will be critically assessed within this chapter, drawing on research from the fields of health policy, health economics, and medical sociology, in addition to STS studies of 'promissory discourses'. The chapter begins with a very brief outline of the developments in the field of genetics and geomics up to and including the HGP.[1]

[1] 'Personalised' rather than 'Precision' will be the preferred term used in this chapter to describe pharmacogenomic-based medicine. This is because of this term's close association with the original 'promissory-vision' for a post-genomic medicine (see Theory Box 6.1).

I. Crinson, *The Biomedical Sciences in Society*,
https://doi.org/10.1007/978-981-15-9523-3_6

From Mendelian Genetics to Molecular Genomics: A Brief Journey

Molecular biology, the study of macromolecules and the macromolecular mechanisms in living organisms, has its origins in the 1930s, but it was Watson and Crick's delineation of the double helix structure of DNA in 1953 that set the stage for the exponential developments that have occurred in the field of genetics and genomics over the past half century. From the development of recombinant DNA (see Glossary) techniques in the 1970s to the genome sequencing projects of the 1990s, new methods and research instruments have proliferated within the science.

These developments in the science of genomics represented a fundamental shift from the classic Mendelian understanding of genes as non-observable 'units of heritability'. In classic genetics, heritability was never precisely conceptualised, but rather followed the notion that, like inheriting the parental home and wealth, a person acquired the features and personalities of their family through their genes. Molecular genetics is no longer concerned with prediction and causality in accounting for individual difference, but with understanding the biochemical processes and structures involved in heritability. This transition brought with it an emphasis on the continuity of the life cycle rather than that at a single point of individual heredity. This is the idea that living things are objects with continuity in space and time:

> *The different organisms we identify as the ancestors of a given individual over successive generations are recurrent patterns in a continuing life cycle of changes, and what part of the life cycle will count as "the organism" should be considered as no more than an arbitrary decision...(therefore), if living things are life cycles, it is natural to ask not merely what DNA does during reproduction and development, but what it does all the time, and what role it plays as a part of the continuously functioning cells that are parts of larger organic systems*. (Barnes and Dupré 2008: 49)

Yet molecular biology has also introduced elements of scientific reductionism, these are seen to manifest themselves at two very distinct levels, the methodological and the ontological. Methodological reductionism is reflected in the view that 'the most fruitful investigative strategy is the decomposition of systems into their component parts', while ontological reductionism is the philosophical assumption (common to the biosciences) that all 'living systems are exhaustively composed of physical components' (Griffiths and Stotz 2013: 58). Here it should be noted that although a molecular identity of the gene was firmly established, a thorough-going Kuhnian paradigmatic revolution did not occur in molecular genetics. Some of the core instrumental ideas associated with Mendelian gene continue to persist to this today within the sub-field of genomics known as behavioural genetics.

The 1980s saw molecular genetics move into it was has been described as its first reductionist phase in attempting to understand the basis of living systems. Genes came to be seen not as unitary holistic objects, but as mere four-letter sequences of DNA. If genes are identified as material objects at all, then this is as composite and spatially discontinuous objects (this more integrative approach was to eventually became known as systems biology and is outlined in detail in Chap. 3). A single gene may now plausibly be identified as DNA, but an entire set of genes cannot be thought of as so many separate pieces of DNA, each of which constitute the substrate of one of the genes. So that, for example, 'the-gene-for' cystic fibrosis can be any of over a thousand DNA sequences known to code for functionally defective variants of the implicated protein, so it is hardly a well-defined object. The shift of 'ontological authority' (see Glossary) from whole gene-based theories to DNA-based theories and chemical-molecular models of structure and function is what marks the divide between genomics and traditional genetics (Barnes and Dupré 2008: 59). More recent developments in molecular bioscience have further begun to erode the once strongly held position that genes are the basic building blocks in all biological processes:

> *There being more to inheritance than nuclear DNA...although all biomolecules are ultimately synthesised from a nucleic acid template, that template is only one source of the specificity of these biomolecules...the specific roles played by the gene in its several identities are more than enough to explain its central place in biology. There is no need for anything more grandiose.* (Griffiths and Stotz 2013: 8)

Sequencing the Human Genome and Its Aftermath

The case for sequencing the human genome was first made in the 1980s on the basis that it would accelerate biomedical research and provide the tools to further a better understanding of the mechanisms and causes of human disease. This objective would become encapsulated within what was to become the Human Genome Project (HGP). The goals of the HGP were first articulated in 1988 by a special committee of the US National Academy of Sciences (NAS), and later adopted through a detailed series of five-year plans jointly written by the US National Institutes of Health and the US Department of Energy. However, it was soon realised that achieving this massive undertaking would require collaboration with research institutes across the world. Hence the formation of what became the International Human Genome Sequencing Consortium (IHGSC), which included the involvement of the Wellcome Trust Institute based in Cambridge (today the site of The Wellcome Trust Genome Campus). In June 2000, the IHGSC announced the availability of a rough draft of the human genome sequence, and in April 2003, the final version was published. The completed sequencing produced the surprise finding that there were only approximately 20,000 human genes, about the same number as a starfish. The function of the remaining 95% of the human genome remained unknown at the time and was labelled evolutionary 'junk'. Since this time, it has been found that this remaining DNA plays an important role in regulating the genome.

When the original funding for the HGP was announced back in 1990, it was claimed that sequencing the human genome would provide the information that would enable clinical practice to move from an era of 'mass health' to the individual 'customisation' of medicine (Dumit 2012: 8). Billions of research dollars have been spent on genome-wide association studies (GWAS) following completion of HGP, but this research had managed to identify only a disappointing number of gene variants of genuine significance for human health given the initially high levels of expectation (Tutton 2016: 1). In this early post-HGP period, or 'post-genomic era' as it has become widely known, it became evident that much higher levels of genotype variation occurred across populations than had been initially assumed. It followed that studying the genome of small numbers of individuals would be insufficient for the understanding of the relationship of our genes to health and disease outcomes. By 2010, it was clear that in order to achieve the translational goal of drawing upon genomic information for future clinical diagnostic and therapeutic interventions, it would be necessary to scale-up research programmes to sequence the genomic make-up of hundreds of thousands of individuals. It also became clear that for a medicine built on genomic profiling to become viable, then the genomic information of individuals had to be linked to their personal social and medical history.

It was these considerations that provided the basis for the establishment of population-based genomic sequencing programmes in a number of high-income countries. Some of these national programmes focused on single diseases, while others were more broad-based. Some programmes did not allow for a capability of returning results to participants, while others plan for whole genome sequencing with a return of results to participants and health care providers. In the UK, 'Genome England' was established by the Department of Health in 2013, with the goal of sequencing 100,000 genomes from NHS patients with rare diseases and their families, as well as patients with common cancers. One of the explicit targets of this programme was to kick start the development of a UK genomics industry. The target of sequencing 100,000 genomes was achieved in December 2018, and as a result, the UK government announced plans to expand the Project in order to sequence 1 million whole genomes by the NHS and UK Biobank within five years. The USA was slightly behind the curve in establishing a similar research programme. It was not until 2015 that President Barack Obama made the announcement that the USA would embark on a government-funded initiative, entitled the 'All of Us Program'. Its objective was to enrol over one million participants who would be expected to share their personal data generated or captured over a period of ten years or more. This data would be sourced from sequencing programmes, electronic medical records, personally reported information, and digital health technologies. The goal of the Program was not only to drive the understanding of disease biology and pathogenesis, but also to constitute the informational basis for developing 'precision-driven' (see Glossary) health care for individuals and populations (Ginsburg and Philips 2018: 694). The programme finally opened for enrolment in May 2018, and as of July 2019 more than 175,000 participants had contributed 'biospecimens' (Denny et al. 2019).

As population-wide genomic data has become available, so an increasing number of pharmacogenomic biomarkers (concerned with gene-drug response associations) of individual drug efficacy have been isolated, and recommendations for their therapeutic use have been published. However, the uptake of 'personalised' medicine has been highly variable in health care systems; 'even when their actionability has been supported by evidence' (Ginsburg and Philips 2018:

696). A recent literature review of the implementation of genomic science into practical therapeutics concluded that, 'although genomic discovery provides the potential for population health benefit, the current knowledge base around implementation to turn this promise into a reality is severely limited' (Roberts et al. 2017: 860). If the much heralded genomic revolution in the delivery of health care is to happen, then one essential requirement is to broaden the average clinician's knowledge of pharmacogenomics (NHS Genomics Education Programme 2018).

▶ **Theory Box 6.1 Promissory Discourses and the Sociology of Expectations** In recent years, there has been an analytical interest within STS-based research in what are described as 'promissory discourses'. The notion of 'discourse' being a standardised concept within constructionist social and philosophical theory, of which STS studies constitutes an important element. The now widespread application of this concept is usually attributed to the French philosopher, Michel Foucault, who recognised 'discourse' as an institutionalised way of structuring and elucidating a particular understanding of reality.

For Foucault, discourses do not arise spontaneously, but are produced by effects of power within a given social order, and this power prescribes the particular rules and categories for what counts as legitimate knowledge and truth about some aspect of the social world. In short, discourses provide a framework that defines what can be thought and said about the world. As such, discourses are social constructions, and the 'promissory discourses' of science are those representations constructed by scientists associated with their attempt to translate 'promising' research findings into funded research projects.

As Borup et al. (2006) have argued, 'novel technologies and fundamental changes in scientific principle do not substantively pre-exist themselves, except and only in terms of the imaginings, expectations and visions that have shaped their potential. As such, future-oriented abstractions are among the most important objects of enquiry for scholars and analysts of innovation' (2006: 285). Positive expectations about the predicted benefits of research are an absolute requirement in securing the support of government and other major funders necessary to develop the research infrastructures that can realistically deliver on said promises. Some better known examples of promissory discourses in biomedical science include programmes in stem cell research, xenotransplantation, gene therapy, nanotechnologies, and pharmacogenomics.

Although the everyday use of the term 'expectations' refers to a state of looking forward, within STS, expectations are conceptualised as 'real-time representations of future technological situations and capabilities…(which) stress that expectations are wishful enactments of a desired future. By performing such futures, they are made real and it is in this sense that expectations can be understood as performative' (Borup et al. 2006: 286). This quote references the notion of 'performativity', a key organising principle within Actor Network Theory-informed STS research. It can be understood as 'the dynamic moves and circular processes whereby presentation, language and bodies of knowledge co-constitute the realities they ostensibly describe' (Latour 2005).

It is through these performative practices that a 'reality', a future vision for a particular socio-technological innovation, is constructed: 'a practice of handling, intervening in the world and thereby enacting one of its versions, up to bringing it into bring' (Mol and Law 2006: 19). The performativity of research science expectations is seen to bridge or mediate across the boundaries separating scientists, investors, and governmental regulatory actors, so constituting an innovation network representing mutually binding obligations and agendas.

A Promissory Vision for Pharmacogenomics and the Role of Big Pharma

Promissory visions (see Theory Box 6.1) and the role they play in building the basis for the funding and delivering of the political support necessary to sustain innovative scientific research programmes and innovation is a crucial one. Richard Tutton has argued that personalised medicine is a particularly pertinent example of the expectations that are associated with such visions:

> '(It) encapsulates both the excesses of promissory science and the inevitable disappointments and disputes that follow. Those who were once hopeful or excited in the 1990s by the prospects of what would be achieved by genomics are now less certain…. (P)ersonalised medicine is therefore an appealing yet ambiguous and contested term and is as such an ideal one for engaging with the claims and counterclaims about the value of genomics to biomedicine' (Tutton 2014: 3).

It was the growing concern with the effects of drug toxicity linked to patented over-the-counter medicines that was the primary reason for the introduction of legislation to regulate the manufacture and use of medicines both in the USA and in the UK at the end of the nineteenth century. By the mid-twentieth century, with a significant increase in both the numbers of pharmaceuticals available and the numbers of people consuming them, reports of adverse drug reactions (ADRs) were beginning to climb steadily. By the early 1970s, drug reactions constituted one of the top ten causes of hospitalisation in the USA. The science behind what would eventually to become pharmacogenomics was established precisely in order to better understand this individual variation in drug responsiveness. The initial work in this field was conducted in the USA in 1950s and early 1960s by Kalow, Motulsky, and Vogel who were concerned with developing a genetic explanation of drug reactions, what they termed 'pharmacological individuality'. However, this research on the heritable pattern of drug responses and enzyme metabolism ultimately became side-tracked by a particular concern with the question of racial difference in drug response. Motulsky later conceded that it was difficult to separate genetic from environmental factors and that few drug responses could be associated with a single gene (Tutton 2014: 46).

By the 1970s, the pharmaceutical industry was still reluctance to admit the extent of genetic variation between patients and its effect on drug response and so had little incentive to conduct research into the avoidance of ADRs. As late as 1999, a paper in *Nature Biotechnology* suggested that the attitudes of executives at big pharmaceutical companies towards genomics and its relevance for their business ranged from 'ignorance to ambivalence' (Regalado 1999: 46—cited in Tutton 2014). Nevertheless, the 1980s saw a gradual recognition of the potentiality of utilising recombinant DNA techniques to develop new kinds of therapeutic products, including monoclonal antibodies (see Glossary), hormones, and blood products, did began to attract funding within the industry. An important factor in this change of direction by Big Pharma was the challenge it now appeared to face from the growth of a new biotechnology industries sector in the economy, promoting its own promissory vision of personalised pharmacogenomics-based medicine. This was a vision that was fostered and funded by government and venture capital, both in the UK and in the USA, from the early 1990s onwards (Hedgecoe and Martin 2003). There was now a clear sense that an understanding of genomic variation could be capitalised upon in order to generate economic value for the new biotechnology companies and Big Pharma alike. In his study of these biotechnology start-ups, Rajan (2006) uses the expression 'venture science' to describe the ways in which these companies sold a vision of the future to generate capital in the present. This was essential in an industry where the developmental pipeline is a long one, often a decade or more, requiring them to 'sell visions of their future products as much as or more than selling the products themselves' (2006: 129).

By the beginning of this century, the term 'pharmacogenomics' (PGx) was being widely used to describe the science involved in identifying the processes by which DNA variants in an individual's genome can increase or decrease the effectiveness of particular medicines. As such, PGx was also being hailed as the potential solution to the 'crisis' of profitability faced by the pharmaceutical industry at this time. This 'crisis' reflected the increasingly longer lead times required for new products to reach the market, combined with the rising development costs, all of which directly impacted on levels of profit-making. The industry proponents of PGx asserted that it could improve productivity as drug development would henceforth require smaller trials and shorter lead times for production, as well as having the potential to make existing products more effective (all three of these promissory visions were subsequently shown to be flawed). A paper published by the pharmaceutical firm Abbott Laboratories at this time (in 2001) concluded that the average efficacy rate of what it termed 'undisclosed major drugs' was just 51%. The paper claimed that PGx could radically improve this efficacy rate by differentiating patients into two groups, those who are more likely to show an efficacious response than the population as a whole, and those who are less likely. This would lead to a better understanding of the risk-to-benefit ratio of any particular drug (Spear et al. 2001: 201—cited in Tutton 2014).

Since the 1950s, the efficacy of pharmaceuticals has been assessed through randomised control trials (RCTs), but this methodology is only able to demonstrate group not individual results. That is, RCTs could predict whether the average patient will gain (or not) a therapeutic benefit from a particular drug but could not predict which patients will definitely benefit or who will react adversely. Pharmacogenetic RCTs were presented as an improvement over traditional RCT approaches on the basis that they were able to measure the independent effects of the genotype, the drug response, and the gene-drug interaction in the active drug and placebo/control groups: '(It) becomes possible to distinguish the differences between simple markers of disease progression and true pharmacogenetic markers, whose effect on disease progression is only seen in the presence of a drug' (Ross et al. 2012: 5). However, a major limitation of pharmacogenomics RCTs is the cost and time required to conduct these studies, requiring as they do a large sample size to provide sufficient statistical power to detect even a modest effect size.

One cogent view of the 'crisis' in the pharmaceutical industry at the beginning of the twenty-first century was that productivity had nothing to do with the time it took to produce successful drugs but rather the lack of therapeutic innovation in the industry. The evidence for this view comes from data produced by the US Food and Drug Administration's (FDA) Center for Drug Evaluation and Research (CDER), which classifies certain drugs for review as new molecular entities (NMEs). NMEs are drugs that have not previously appeared in an approval application and as such qualify for priority in the FDA review process: 'Many of these products contain active moieties (see Glossary) that have not been approved by FDA previously, either as a single ingredient drug or as part of a combination product; these products frequently provide important new therapies for patients' (FDA 2015). Between 1989 and 2000, the FDA gave priority status to just 15% of the total number of drugs it approved. This is evidence that the business model of the pharmaceutical industry in this period was primarily about turning-out minor variants of existing approved drugs ('next-in-class'), and the development of so-called 'blockbuster drugs' that exceeded $1 Billion in Global sales. Examples of the latter were Ranitidine (trade name Zantac) for the treatment of stomach ulcers, this was followed by Fluoxetine (trade name—Prozac) for depressive disorders and Sildenafil (trade name—Viagra) for erectile dysfunction.

The tension between this profitable business model and those who were urging the industry to invest in the science of PGx was clear. Personalised genomic-based drugs challenged the very idea of 'one-size-fits-all' blockbuster drugs, but Big Pharma had no intention of either narrowing their market or their profit margins in the early years of the twenty-first century.

The Challenge of Integrating a Personalised Medicine Within Health Care Systems

The history of personalisation within medical practice long predates that of the potential attributed to pharmacogenomics. Throughout the course of the nineteenth century, as modern medicine began to gradually progress towards developing new classificatory systems of disease diagnosis and with that a greater effectiveness in the managing of illness, it was only wealthy individuals that had direct access to this burgeoning medical expertise. If only by default, the practice of medicine at this point in history was individualised. The term 'personal medicine' also origins in another period of history, the 1930s, being associated with a social movement that sought to promote a more holistic ('patient-as-person') approach to diagnosis and treatment. This was in reaction to a perceived 'once-size-fits-all' approach emergent from the new developments in what was described as 'mass medicine'. Personalised medicine was seen as being able to take account of a patient's social background and their unique biographies; this was an explicit critique of the direction taken by clinical practice which it was argued was leading to 'de-personalisation' of the individual patient.

But greater clinical efficacy became the popular demand for widening access to medical care for the majority of the population on the basis of their health need not their income. The mid-twentieth century saw the gradual introduction of universal health care systems across the world (with the notable exception of the USA), and the adoption of population-level approaches to disease prediction and management. Yet by the turn of the century, these strategies were being presented, particularly in the USA, as having failed to fulfil their promise of 'health for all'. This highly politicised discourse concerning the future direction of health care was the background to the construction of a promissory vision for a 'return' to a personalised system of medicine, building on the early developments in pharmacogenomics. This twenty-first-century promissory vision envisages a transformation in the way the doctors manage the care of individual patients, facilitated by the tools of PGx and focused on the individual genotype. With this information at hand, it was argued that clinicians would be better placed to predict the likely response of their patient's to a recommended course of drug treatment for a given condition before the drug was actually administered. If it was determined that a patient was susceptible to an adverse drug reaction or if the drug treatment was unlikely to be efficacious based on the genomic and personal information, then an alternative personalised drug treatment can then be prescribed.

The introduction of pharmacogenomic pre-testing would certainly mark a significant departure from the current trial-and-error approach to drug prescribing. In theory it would enable a clinician to predict which of their patients were likely to experience ADRs. In turn, this would reduce the number of hospitalisations required to treat drug side-effects with a commensurate saving for health care providers. In a private insurance-based health care system such as the USA, this is very much a pertinent issue with the potential to reduce (or increase) an individual's health insurance premiums. In the general taxation-funded 'single payer' National Health System in the UK, ADRs constituted approximately 6% of all admissions which equated to 4% of hospital bed capacity in 2014 (RPS 2014). While in 2018, one report estimated that avoidable ADRs consumed 181,626 bed-days in the NHS, a direct cause in 712 deaths, and contributing to a further 1708 deaths (Elliott et al. 2018). Therefore, the cost savings to the British state, where in 2020 total health expenditure (THE) amounted to over £200 billion, or nearly 10% of GDP, are potentially considerable.

The development of the first large-scale epidemiological cohort studies in the 1950s established the now familiar research approach to understanding the social patterns of disease, generating statistical correlations between known health 'risk factors' and the incidence of disease in a particular population. What become known as the risk assessment process sought to link these identifiable risk factors, primarily conceived as volitional health behaviours, directly with actual or potential harm. It was on this basis that health risk came to be seen almost as if it were the disease itself. In the USA, pharmaceutical companies were by the 1980s already engaging in direct-to-consumer (DTC) advertising to make individuals aware of a disease for which they were potentially 'at risk', through self-diagnosis checklists. 'Personalising' increasingly meant that the 'possibility of risk in general now becomes your possible risk' (Dumit 2012: 65). At this point it is worth remembering the injunction of the eminent British public health academic Geoffrey Rose that 'all interventions should be based on absolute measures of risk; relative risk is strictly for researchers only' (1992: 152).

In terms of the process of developing actual 'personalised' drugs, one of the first and still one of the most famous is Herceptin. The drug was approved in 1998 by the FDA, for the treatment of metastatic breast cancer in women with tumours that over-express the HER2 protein, simultaneously with a companion diagnostic called 'HercepTest' to determine which patients with these tumours were suitable for treatment. Herceptin was also therefore the first example of what became known as a 'combination product', meaning that a drug could not be prescribed without the genomic test first being administered. The crucial difference with conventional chemotherapy for breast cancer was that Herceptin left non-cancerous cells unaffected so avoiding many of the usual side-effects. It is significant that this drug, which is often cited as the exemplar of the personalised medicine 'revolution', was never at the time described as such by its manufacturer. This was on the scientific basis that only genotype should be used to segregate responding from non-responding patients. In the case of Herceptin, the companion test for HER2 overexpression measures a phenotype, a specific protein defect, that is not directly linked to genotype (Haseltine 1998: 885—cited in Tutton 2014). The genotype-phenotype separation represents the difference between 'somatic mutations' (see Glossary) in the genomes of tumours growing inside patients and their inherited genome. Over the subsequent 20 years, cancer research has focused on developing new targeted treatments directed at the phenotypic mutations present in the tumour DNA, but not the within the germline. It is these targeted drugs that are today seen as exemplars of PGx.

Today, Herceptin is now rarely prescribed as a monotherapy and is generally used alongside conventional chemotherapy. The usual side-effects apply to the latter, but evidence that Herceptin itself produces ADRs has also started to grow. The drug has though been a huge financial success for its manufacturer, which would suggest that profit can be generated from a personalised drug (albeit that Herceptin does not quite fit the standard definition) effective only for a minority of patients diagnosed with breast cancer. The example of Herceptin and other personalised medicines such as Ziagen, used as part of an antiretroviral combination therapy to treat HIV, shows that while PGx is able to produce new sets of statistical probabilities that aim to refine which groups of patients will gain therapeutic benefit or avoid ADRs, it still cannot precisely identify who will benefit or not. On this basis PGx cannot be seen as a panacea to eradicate adverse reactions or make all drugs efficacious (Tutton 2014: 83).

A key marker of the advance towards accessible personalised medicine would be the number of PGx combined treatments that have been approved for use by the FDA, and in the UK by the European Medicines Agency. However this is rather more complex a test than would appear at first sight. In 2011, the FDA produced guidance that stated, '(it) supported the development of therapeutic products that *depend on* the use of approved or cleared IVD (in vitro diagnostics) companion diagnostic devices, and that ideally a therapeutic product and its corresponding companion diagnostic device would be developed *contemporaneously*' (FDA 2011—emphasis *not* in original). Up until this time, the FDA had only approved three such combination products of drugs and diagnosis (one of which was Herceptin). Beyond the approval of new drugs the FDA has made inserting PGx data in drug labels the central part of its strategy to support the development of this technology. The objective being to identify opportunities to update product labels with DNA variant information on already marketed drugs (in some instances decades after first approval), in order to make the use of already marketed drugs safer and effective. And secondly, to include the PGx data on drug labels as a means of disseminating information even when this is not directly relevant to clinical treatment decisions (Tutton 2014: 89). By 2019, the FDA had included such information on 267 previously approved drugs (FDA 2019). Yet at the same time very few next-generation combination therapies have been approved by the FDA and come onto the market.

The limited development of new PGx therapeutics poses questions about the economic business model adopted by the major pharmaceutical companies that place potential profitability before health need in drug research development investment decisions. The market for combination therapies are those groups identified as being at high risk, which by definition means the numbers are going to be small; certainly not the mass market for 'one-size-fits-all' blockbuster drugs. One of the reasons for the more recent use of the term 'precision' rather than 'personalised' medicine is that the latter term is actually better suited to describing the business model of Amazon than an accurate description of a PGx model for therapeutics. Amazon 'personalises' or targets their goods and services based on individual demographics, previous purchases, and recommendations from 'friends'. Yet even for Amazon, this marketing approach has never been about the unique selling of goods to a 'personalised' customer, but rather what has been termed 'mass customisation', where individuals with shared interests and preferences are grouped together (Piller and Tseng 2010:

7—cited in Tutton 2014). Manufacturing companies do not generally make individual items that will be purchased by only one person, and this is certainly the case for Big Pharma, where the economics of the manufacturing process would mitigate against bespoke production. At best, delivering on the promise of 'personalised medicine' for pharmaceutical companies would mean following the mass customisation model and grouping patients into shared genotypes to achieve the economies of scale necessary for profitability.

In contemporary health care systems in high-income economies, clinicians increasingly no longer enjoy the autonomy to determine what constitutes the most efficient and effective therapeutics for their patients. Regulatory agencies such as the FDA in the USA and the EMA in Europe exist to approve drugs and medical devices on the basis of their safety and efficacy. Several national health care systems also have a further layer of regulation. In the UK, the National Institute for Health and Clinical Excellence (abbreviated as NICE) was first established in 1999 as an 'arms-length' body (from government) to evaluate the evidence for the clinical efficacy *and* the cost-effectiveness of both new and existing 'health technologies'. This evaluation process is carried out at the request of the Department of Health, and the responsibility for determining the efficacy and effectiveness of new therapies now resides with specialised health technology appraisal (HTA) panels. These appraisal panels usually consist of biomedical scientists, clinical specialists, as well as representatives of relevant patient groups. As Tutton points out in his summary of the interviews he carried out with senior NICE committee members; 'HTA focuses on the management of groups of patients as opposed to an individual in the case of personalised medicine…the pharmaceutical industry has never liked HTA, it prefers to have just three hurdles to jump, quality, safety and efficacy, and not a fourth one, cost effectiveness' (2014: 105). The cost-effectiveness of new therapeutics has been assessed by NICE HTA panels since their inception, on the basis of a measure that derives from health economics known as a QALY (quality-adjusted life year). The QALY formulae used by NICE limits spending on therapeutics to a life year gained for a maximum threshold cost. Over the past two decades, there have been many examples of efficient conventional medicines being refused approval for use on the grounds of lack of cost-effectiveness for the public-funded NHS (Crinson 2004: 32). On the basis of this approach, most PGx combined therapies would not be cost-effective as they involve both the costs of testing followed by drug treatment. The high cost of these therapies is also problematic in private insurance-based systems such as the USA and the social insurance systems of many countries within Europe and elsewhere that set limits to the cost reimbursement to patients of such therapies.

In addition to the high costs of combined therapies, there are other barriers to the design and implementation of a strategy to deliver pharmacogenomic personalisation without contradicting the key organising principles of health care systems that are characterised by 'universal coverage' (see Glossary), such as the NHS in the UK. The ideal would be for a pre-emptive strategy to be adopted by the health care system that would involve a process of screening to generate variant data for multiple pharmacogenes for individual patients, before prescription of any target drug for that individual. The data on variant DNA would then be included in the individual's Electronic Health Record (EHR) which could be linked to clinical decision-making support to provide the necessary specialist advice if prescribing a target drug to that individual patient. The complexities of such an approach are clear, requiring as they do, 'extensive curation of the pharmacogenomic evidence, expert design of the pharmacogenomic test, curation of predicted consequences of the genetic variants, clinical expertise regarding drug prescribing and alternatives, and technical expertise to support laboratory testing, reporting, and decision support' (Roden et al. 2019: 528). The decision taken in 2010 by the UK Department of Health to abandon the construction of a nationally integrated Electronic Patient Record system, budgeted to cost £12bn and said to be the largest civilian IT programme in the world system at the time, demonstrates the difficulties of establishing the necessary infrastructure for an effective and efficient information system able to realise individualised PGx-based health care.

As an illustration of the difficulties associated with adopting a personalised medicine-based approach within health care practice, let us look at the management of a patient with cancer as one example. The therapeutic ideal would be for a molecular analysis of a tumour in an individual patient to be carried out, this would enable the selection of an effective drug(s) to control its growth and prolong survival. This approach is appealing to both cancer patient groups and charities that support cancer research. However, there remains a lack of clarity about the therapeutic benefit of such an approach: '(T)here should also be a clear message to patients that personalized cancer medicine has not led to gains in survival or its quality and is an appropriate strategy only within well-designed clinical trials' (Tannock and Hickman 2016: 1289).

The vision of PGx becoming a day-to-day reality in health care systems, an essential tool for patient diagnosis and care, also requires the support and commitment of front line professionals, including both clinicians and pharmacists. The STS literature has provided many examples of research pointing to the difficulties faced by laboratory-based scientists in persuading clinicians that new innovations are actually relevant and useful for their practice (some of these examples are discussed in Chap. 3). This in part reflects the different epistemic cultures in play and relies on scientists being able to convince clinicians that their current patient management practices are in some way problematic or deficient. In the case of delivering a personalised medicine, this would also require the support of pharmacogenomic specialists able to provide the support for clinicians in interpreting the results of PGx testing (van der Wouden 2017: 341). A lack of clinician knowledge and awareness of PGx, particularly in primary care provision in the UK, is often frequently cited as a barrier to adoption. Many clinicians who completed their training over a decade ago would have had little to no genomic medicine included in their medical school curriculum. Additionally, 'technology and discoveries in genomics have advanced at tremendous speed, making it very difficult to stay updated on all the novel opportunities. Although the scientific evidence and clinical benefit of PGx is strong, it can all remain unclear due to poor literacy in genomics, which lowers the overall acceptance' (Krebs and Milani 2019: 6).

The variable implementation of PGx within clinical practice is not simply a question of a perceived professional-cultural resistance or genomic knowledge deficits. There is also a lack of clear evidence concerning the efficaciousness of PGx testing for day-to-day clinical practice uptake (Rafi et al. 2020). In conclusion then: '(P)recision medicine and the ecosystem that supports it, must embrace patient centeredness and engagement, digital health, genomics and other molecular technologies, data sharing and data science to be successful' (Ginsburg and Philips 2018: 694). It also has to be in tune with the principles of universalism that define the delivery of care in the majority of health care systems across the globe. In these systems, scare health care resources have to be equitably distributed, and the relatively limited evidence for the cost-effectiveness of PGx-based medicine has slowed its uptake; this evidence is only now slowly emerging (Krebs and Milani 2019: 3).

An Era of Personal Genomics?

Post-HGP, the possibility of using associations found to exist between genetic variants and disease risk to build individual 'genome profiles' slowly began to be realised. For nearly two decades both industry and academic genomic scientists have working together in order to establish publically available reference databases on the 4–5 million single nucleotide polymorphisms (SNP). SNPs are the most common type of genetic variation and occur normally throughout a person's DNA. These variations may be unique or occur in many individuals, and it is on that understanding that more than 100 million SNPs have been found in populations around the world. Most commonly, 'these variations are found in the DNA between genes. They can act as biological markers, helping scientists locate genes that are associated with disease. When SNPs occur within a gene or in a regulatory region near a gene, they may play a more direct role in disease by affecting the gene's function' (National Institutes of Health—'What are SNP's).

As it gradually began to be recognised that significant genotype variation occurred across populations, so that the establishment of global SNP databases was seen to be a necessary step in order to gain a purchase on individual variability and predisposition to disease. Once the databases began to be built, they opened up the possibilities for genome-wide association studies (GWAS). GWAS are in principle hypothesis-free methods that seek to examine SNPs across the genome in the study of common but complex diseases, where many genetic variations can contribute to individual's risk of that disease. As of January 2020, the online database, 'GWAS Central', identifies 70,566,447 associations between 3,251,694 unique SNPs and 1451 disease/phenotype descriptions (www.gwascentral.org), while the European Bioinformatics Institute GWAS catalogue contains 4628 separate studies (EBI: accessed June 2020). This is a remarkable achievement, given that it was only as far back as 2003 that the US National Human Genome Research Institute (NHGRI) first published its vision for the application of GWAS to develop an individualised preventative medicine initiative.

It was also around this period that the first references to a 'personal genomics' were being made, reflecting a move away from the original 'one-genome-fits-all' assumption of the HGP, in which the DNA from just a few individuals was deemed to be sufficient to explain disease susceptibility. Although the commercial potential of individual genomic testing was recognised by the emergent biotechnology industry in the early 1990s, it was not until a decade or so later, post-HGP, that the innovation of 'gene chips' (see Glossary) enabled individual diagnostic genomic testing to became commercially viable. Relatively small start-up companies were then able to begin to offer direct-to-consumer (DTC) genomic screening services. The cost of DTC services became increasingly affordable as the gene-chip microarrays could be used on desktop machines. This technology, together with sequencing machines and the appropriate reagents, enabled screening for multiple SNPs in parallel. Overtime the capacity of these chips has grown, and today are able to genotype between 500,000 and 5 million SNPs (NHGRI 2019).

As a consumer service, DTC or private genetic testing seeks to use the language of personal choice, empowerment, and self-knowledge to win over new customers. All that is required of the 'consumer', once they have paid their fee, is to provide a brief familial medical history and a saliva sample from which their DNA can be extracted. The results of the SNP analysis are then compared to the variants in the published literature. A statistical association with certain disease states is searched for drawing on GWAS, and the customer is provided with their average lifetime relative risk of a particular disease occurring. A 2019 survey of the DTC industry indicated that there were currently 32 firms marketing 'personalised medicine' genomic testing services globally on the Internet (ISOGG 2019). This number represents a significant drop from a decade previously when some 60 companies were active in promoting 'empowerment' through providing individualised genomic information. Three of the more well-known players were 23andMe, deCODE Genetics, and Navigenics (the latter ceased as a DTC company in 2012). When these DTC companies commenced commercial activities in and around 2007, few large-scale GWAS have been published in the genomics literature. And, while these personal genomics companies were not the first to offer DTC genetic testing, they were the first to monetise the information drawn from the GWAS.

However, for all the developments that have occurred in genomic science, GWAS cannot be relied upon to predict with certainty the likelihood of disease occurring for individuals who use commercial DTC services. This uncertainty is combined with the limited availability of pharmacogenomics knowledge and services available in local health services (described above) when the individual user of a DTC service seeks reassurance and treatment from their own doctor following receipt of their personalised the health risk profile. Concerns have been voiced by many health care regulators, policy advisors, clinicians, and biomedical scientists who were sceptical that 'far from being empowered, users of DTC services would suffer anxiety and make inappropriate use of finite healthcare resources' (Tutton 2016: 4). Yet despite initial enthusiasm from the public, particularly in the USA, the DTC commercial disease-testing balloon slowly deflated over the course of its first decade of existence.

In response, some of the original DTC companies have successfully re-orientated their services towards the marketisation of genealogical or 'ancestry' services.

While the ever-expanding GWAS database has matured into an efficient and effective tool for mapping SNPs that can be reliably associated with a variety of human phenotypes, there remain some important limitations. SNP-based genome testing does not diagnose the presence or absence of a disease in an individual: 'By their very definition, they are forward-looking services that render statistically the probability an individual faces of a disease developing in their lifetime' (Tutton 2014: 129). The absolute lifetime risk calculation provided for each DTC customer does not represent their individualised risk per se, but the average risk for a group that shares a specific genetic variant associated with the onset of a particular disease and the same socio-demographic characteristics. While it is often claimed that the methodology of GWAS is 'hypothesis free', it is based on a set of assumptions known as the 'common disease/common variant' hypothesis. This hypothesis is one that assumes that common diseases can be explained with reference to common variants, which are attributable to relatively common SNPs that have a frequency of 1–5% in the population. However, there is an alternative hypothesis that states that multiple rare variants cause disease at high prevalence in a population. This occurs through a genetic heterogeneity of variants in a single gene or multiple rare variants within genes in the same pathway that have cumulative effects. While the GWAS approach has the statistical power to detect common variants with modest effects, it is less effective at testing rare variation (Monsinger-Reif et al. 2013).

Finally, a paper in *Nature* points to a fundamental biological factor that limits progress towards understanding disease mechanisms; this is the 'difficulty in assigning molecular function to the vast majority of GWAS hits that do not affect protein-coding sequence' (Fahr et al. 2015: 337). This references the role played by the epigenetic process, the way in which a gene may change as a result of little known or uncertain environmental influences. If biomedical science can in the future begin to integrate genetic and epigenetic data then a more nuanced complexity to disease variant function might emerge, but this 'will continue to push the limits of experimental and computational approaches' (Fahr et al. 2015: 340). The science of epigenetics is the focus of the following chapter.

Concluding Comments

With the benefit of hindsight it may be somewhat unfair to conclude this chapter by citing from a vision of a post-genomic future that was being discussed two decades ago. However, the quote taken from the popular science journal '*Science*' in 2001, it is a salutary insight into the problems that can be associated with the construction of promissory visions, and engaging in futurology:

> *We are rapidly advancing upon the postgenomic era in which genetic information will have to be examined in multiple health care situations throughout the lives of individuals…in the not-so-distant future children at high risk for coronary artery disease will be identified and*

> *treated to prevent changes in their vascular walls during adulthood. Parents will have the option to be told their carrier status for many recessive diseases before they decide to start a family. For middle-aged and older populations, we will be able to determine risk profiles for numerous late-onset diseases, preferably before the appearance of symptoms, which at least could be partly prevented through dietary or pharmaceutical interventions. In the near future, the monitoring of individual drug response profiles with DNA tests throughout life will be standard practice. Soon, genetic testing will comprise a wide spectrum of different analyses with a host of consequences for individuals and their families.... The tremendous potential for efficient information transfer via the Internet can and should be used to inform the public of the possibilities provided by the genomics era....(R)eaping the fruits of the human genome sequencing project through alleviating the suffering of patients will only be possible if available genetic information is combined with the skilled professionalism of health care workers and ethically solid standards'.* (Peltonen and McKusick 2001: 1229)

While some of these predictions have proved correct, confidence in the ability of genomic bioscience to build upon the findings of the HGP to effect real change in the health status of populations has not yet come to pass. This in part reflects the fact that health care systems have not been able to adapt themselves to incorporate the developments in pharmacogenetics described in this chapter. This is not simply a matter of the training and education of clinicians and pharmacists. The limited resources available to health services, even in high-income countries, to invest in the potential of genomic medicine reflects the more immediate demands of an ageing population living with long-term disability, chronic disease, and heightened susceptibility to common influenza epidemics and more complex pandemics such as Covid-19. GWAS have revolutionised the study of complex human traits by identifying thousands of genetic loci that contribute to susceptibility for a wide range of common diseases, but the revolution in personal genomics has not developed in a way that was once anticipated.

Chapter Summary—Key Points

- *Classic Mendelian genetics was concerned with the understanding of genes as non-observable 'units of heritability'.*
- *Molecular genetics is not concerned with prediction and causality in accounting for individual difference, but with understanding the biochemical processes and structures.*
- *Developments in pharmacogenomics (PGx) have offered a promissory vision of a 'personalised' medicine for the future.*
- *PGx is concerned with identifying the processes by which DNA variants in an individual's genome can increase or decrease the effectiveness of particular medicines.*
- *The development pipeline for biotechnology companies is a long one requiring them to promote future visions of their products that do not always come to fruition.*

- *Pharmacogenomic pre-testing marks a significant departure from the current trial-and-error approach to drug prescribing, enabling ADRs to be avoided in theory.*
- *Big Pharma necessarily puts profitability before population health need in drug development investment decisions.*
- *'Personalised' is less an accurate description of the complexities of the PGx therapeutic model and more accurately describes the business model of the online retailer Amazon.*
- *The market for PGx combination therapies are groups identified as being at high risk, which means they are small in number, not the mass market for 'one-size-fits-all' drugs.*
- *The cost-effectiveness of new therapeutics in the UK is assessed by NICE HTA panels, on the basis of a measure known as a QALY (quality-adjusted life year).*
- *The vision of PGx becoming a day-to-day reality in health care systems, an essential tool for patient diagnosis, requires the support and training of clinicians and pharmacists.*
- *The idea of 'personal genomics' is one that seeks to commercially capitalise on the outcome of extensive GWAS, identifying the role of gene variants in common disease.*
- *DTC or private genetic testing seeks to use the language of personal choice, empowerment, and self-knowledge to win over new customers.*
- *SNP-based genome testing does not diagnose the presence or absence of a disease, rather they state the probability of an individual acquiring a disease over a lifetime.*
- *Far from being empowered, individual users of DTC services potentially suffer anxiety and make inappropriate use of finite conventional healthcare resources.*

Bibliography

Barnes, B., & Dupré, J. (2008). *Genomes and What to Make of Them*. London: University of Chicago Press.

Borup, M., Brown, N., Konrad, K., & Van Lente, H. (2006). The Sociology of Expectations in Science and Technology. *Technological Analysis and Strategic Management, 18*(3), 285–298.

Crinson, I. (2004). The Politics of Regulation within the 'Modernised' NHS: The Case of Beta Interferon & the 'Cost-Effective' Treatment of Multiple Sclerosis. *Critical Social Policy, 24*(1), 30–49.

Denny, J., Rutter, J., Goldstein, D., Philippakis, A., Smoller, J., Jenkins, J., & Dishman, E. (2019). The 'All of US' Research Program. *The New England Journal of Medicine, 381*, 668–676.

Dumit, J. (2012). *Drugs for Life: How Pharmaceutical Companies Define Our Health*. Durham & London: Duke University Press.

Elliott, R., Camacho, E., Campbell, F., Jankovic, D., Martyn St James, M., Kaltenthaler, E., et al. (2018). *Prevalence and Economic Burden of Medication Errors in the NHS in England*. Sheffield. Policy Research Unit in Economic Evaluation of Health & Care Interventions (EEPRU).

Fahr, K. and 20 Other Authors. (2015). Genetic and Epigenetic Fine-Mapping of Causal Autoimmune Disease Variants. *Nature, 518*(7539), 337–343.

FDA. (2011). *Guidance for Industry E16 Biomarkers Related to Drug or Biotechnology Product Development: Context, Structure, and Format of Qualification Submissions*. Silver Springs, MD: US Food and Drug Administration.

FDA. (2015). New Molecular Entity Approvals. Retrieved September 2015, from http://www.fda.gov/Drugs/DevelopmentApprovalProcess/DrugInnovation/ucm336115.htm.

FDA. (2019). Pharmacogenomic Drug Labeling. Retrieved November 2019, from www.fda.gov/drugs/science-and-research-drugs/table-pharmacogenomic-biomarkers-drug-labeling.

Ginsburg, G., & Philips, K. (2018). Precision Medicine from Science to Value. *Health Affairs, 37*(5), 694–701.

Griffiths, P., & Stotz, K. (2013). *Genetics and Philosophy*. Cambridge: Cambridge University Press.

Haseltine, W. (1998). Not Quite Pharmacogenomics. *Nature Biotechnology, 16*, 1295–1296.

Hedgecoe, A., & Martin, P. (2003). The Drugs Don't Work: Expectations and the Shaping of Pharmacogenetics. *Social Studies of Science, 33*, 327–364.

ISOGG - International Society of Genetic Genealogy. (2019). List of Testing Companies. isogg.org/wiki/List_of_DNA_testing_companies – accessed December 2019.

Krebs, K., & Milani, L. (2019). Translating Pharmacogenomics into Clinical Decisions: Do Not Let the Perfect Be the Enemy of the Good. *Human Genomics, 13*, 39.

Latour, B. (2005). *Reassembling the Social: An Introduction to Actor-Network-Theory*. Oxford: Oxford University Press.

Mol, A.-M., & Law, J. (2006). Complexities: An introduction. In J. Law & A.-M. Mol (Eds.), *Complexities: Social Studies of Knowledge Practices* (pp. 1–22). Durham, NC: Duke University Press.

Monsinger-Reif, A., Jorgenson, E., Relling, M., Kroetz, D., Weinshilboum, R., Cox, N. J., & Roden, D. (2013). Genome-Wide Association Studies in Pharmacogenomics: Successes and Lessons. *Pharmacogenet Genomics, 23*(8), 383–394.

National Human Genome Research Institute (NHGRI). (n.d.). Retrieved November 2019, from https://www.genome.gov/about-genomics/.

National Institutes of Health (NIH). (n.d.-a). *What Are Single Nucleotide Polymorphisms (SNPs)?* Retrieved November 2019, from https://ghr.nlm.nih.gov/primer/genomicresearch/snp.

NHS. (2018). Genomics Education Programme. Retrieved September 2019, from www.genomicseducation.hee.nhs.uk.

Peltonen, L., & McKusick, V. (2001). Dissecting Human Disease in the Postgenomic Era. *Science, 291*(5507), 1224–1229.

Piller, F., & Tseng, M. (2010). *Handbook of Research in Mass Customization and Personalization*. New Jersey: World Scientific Books.

Rafi, I., Crinson, I., Dawes, M., Rafi, D., Pirmohamed, M., & Walter, F. M. (2020). The Implementation of Pharmacogenomics into UK General Practice: A Qualitative Study Exploring Barriers, Challenges and Opportunities. *Journal of Community Genetics, 11*(3), 269–277.

Rajan, K. S. (2006). *Biocapital: The Constitution of Postgenomic Life*. Durham & London: Duke University Press.

Regalado, A. (1999). Inventing the Pharmacogenomics Business. *American Journal of Health System Pharma, 56*, 40–50.

Roberts, M., Kennedy, A., Chambers, D., & Khoury, M. (2017). The Current State of Implementation Science in Genomic Medicine: Opportunities for Improvement. *Genetics in Medicine, 19*(8), 858–863.

Roden, D., MacLeod, H., Relling, M., Mensah, G., Peterson, J., & Van Driest, S. (2019). Genomics Medicine 2—Pharmacogenomics. *The Lancet, 394*(10197), 521–532.

Rose, G. (1992). *The Strategy of Preventive Medicine*. Oxford: Oxford University Press.
Ross, S., Anand, S., Joseph, P., & Pare, G. (2012). Promises and Challenges of Pharmacogenetics: An Overview of Study Design, Methodological and Statistical Issues. *JRSM Cardiovascular Disease, 1*, 12.
Royal Pharmaceutical Society. (2014). New Medicines, Better Medicines, Better Use of Medicines. Retrieved from http://www.rpharms.com/promoting-pharmacy-pdfs/nmbmbu%2D%2D-full-report.pdf.
Spear, B., et al. (2001). Clinical Application of Pharmacogenetics. *Trends in Molecular Medicine, 7*, 201–204.
Tannock, I., & Hickman, J. (2016). Limits to Personalised Cancer Medicine. *New England Journal of Medicine, 375*(13), 1289–1294.
Tutton, R. (2014). *Genomics and the Reimagining of Personalized Medicine*. Farnham: Ashgate.
Tutton, R. (2016). Personal Genomics and Its Sociotechnical Transformations. In D. Kumar & R. Chadwick (Eds.), *Genomics and Society* (pp. 1–20). London: Academic Press.
van der Wouden, et al. (2017). Implementing Pharmacogenomics in Europe: Design and Implementation strategy of the Ubiquitous Pharmacogenomics Consortium. *Clinical Pharmacology and Therapeutics, 101*(3), 341–358.

Social Implications of the Epigenetics 'Revolution' 7

Abstract

This chapter critically engages with the field of environmental epigenetics and discusses the social implications of this relatively new field of research. It begins with an outline of the science of epigenetics, moving on to a critical assessment of 'classic' epigenetic studies that link maternal care, stress, and early development to durable long-term behavioural and disease outcomes. It then explores the evidence for both inter- and transgenerational effects of exposure to environmental genomic modifications, often cited as explanations for cycles of poverty and dysfunctional social behaviour. Despite the post-genomic repudiation of 'race' as a biological entity, it continues to be utilised as a variable in environmental epigenetics research. This research will be critically assessed with reference to both research ethics and the appropriate use of proxy measures. The chapter concludes with an assessment of the extent to which environmental epigenetics has opened up the possibility of reconfiguring the long-standing boundary that exists between social and natural science and the prospects for interdisciplinary research.

An Introduction to Epigenetics

In the post-genomic era, epigenetics is increasingly said to be the 'next big thing' in biomedical science. Epigenetics is a heterogeneous field of research that is primarily concerned with understanding the complex mechanisms of cell identity and processes of cell differentiation. This field has acquired a significant public profile, not least because of 'a number of provocative propositions that have caught the attention of the wider public and scientists alike' (Müller et al. 2017: 1677). One such provocative claim being that the study of epigenetics will bring to an end the false dichotomy of nature and nurture in human development!

I. Crinson, *The Biomedical Sciences in Society*,
https://doi.org/10.1007/978-981-15-9523-3_7

Epigenetics has emerged as a 'revolutionary' new framework for conceptualising the material environment that exists outside of the human body as 'bioactive'. This is an understanding of an interactivity between genome and environment that includes factors such as socioeconomic class deprivation, psycho-social factors such as the experience of trauma, as well as exercise habits and nutrition, all are seen as playing a part in influencing biological processes at the molecular level. This emergent understanding also challenges traditional models of health risk that separate 'exterior' risks (to the human body) from 'interior' or genetic risk factors. Environmental epigenetics conceives exterior sources as 'miniaturised environments' and interior sources as molecular and interactive through 'epigenetic logics' (Lloyd and Müller 2018: 676).

The focus on the environment as an epigenetic mechanism of DNA modification has also had the consequence of generating an enthusiasm for interdisciplinary working, with the 'environment' standing as a common denominator at the intersection of the natural sciences, the social sciences, and the humanities. Yet the conception of 'environment' as used within the science of epigenetics is not necessarily coterminous with that referenced by social and environmental scientists. Aside from the cheerleaders for an interdisciplinary epigenetics as offering the potential to expand the understanding of the domain of the 'biosocial', there are those who see the emergence of one form of over-determinism (hereditary genetics) being replaced with another (epigenetic DNA modifications).

This chapter will critically discuss the implications of the findings of this comparatively new field of research for the social and public policy domains. It begins with an outline of the organising principles of epigenetics, before moving on to an assessment of what can be termed 'classic' studies of early neural development. These draw on experimental work with rodents, linking maternal care, stress, and early development to durable long-term behavioural and disease outcomes in humans. The chapter then goes on to explore the evidence for inter- and transgenerational effects of exposure to epigenetic modifiers, which are often cited as an explanation for continuing cycles of poverty and patterns of dysfunctional social behaviour in families. Despite the post-genomic repudiation of the construct of 'race' as a viable biological category of human difference, it continues to be utilised as an independent variable within environmental epigenetics. This research will be critically assessed with reference to ethical concerns as well with the methodology of using proxy measures in bioscience. The chapter concludes with an assessment of the extent to which environmental epigenetics has opened up the possibility of reconfiguring the long-standing epistemic boundary that exists between social and natural science, overcoming the simplistic nature-nurture divide.

Classic Rodent Studies: Stressors and Early Development

The first mention of the term 'epigenetics' was in the 1940s, some time prior to Crick and Watson's discovery of the DNA double helix. It was the preferred term used to describe research that sought to examine the processes through which environmental stimuli interact with genotypes in both individual development and natural selection (Waddington 1942 cited in Pinel et al. 2018). In its post-genomic incarnation, epigenetics is the name given to the field of research concerned with heritable alterations and the processes that control gene expression and regulation that lie beyond DNA sequencing and that are important for normal development and physiology. The 'epigenome' as it is termed comprises all of the chemical compounds which are not part of the DNA sequence, but are on or attached to a person's DNA (genome) as a way to regulate the activity (expression) of all the genes within the genome (NIH 2020).

Epigenetic modifications are understood to regulate gene expression by acting as gatekeepers, blocking or allowing access to a gene's 'on/off' switch. These chemical compounds (such as methyl or acetyl groups) or 'tags' as they are termed are added directly to DNA or on to histones (the large spool-like proteins around which DNA is tightly wound). DNA 'methylation' (see Glossary) masks certain regions on the genome, whereas modifications to histones, termed 'acetylation' (see Glossary), can loosen or tighten the DNA reel, altering which genes are exposed (Wright 2013). Thus the DNA accessibility and the biophysical properties of the chromatin structure (see Glossary) can be altered, thereby effecting patterns of gene expression. Methylation is considered to be a long-term, relatively stable, epigenetic trait, a powerful means by which to suppress the expression of unwanted repetitive or excess genes, so contributing to maintaining the cellular phenotype (Handy et al. 2011: 2145).

While epigenetic processes are crucial to normal development and differentiation, these epigenetic processes can also be modified by environmental and social influences, resulting in the potential alteration of phenotype. This is particularly the case in the early 'critical windows' period of postnatal development. Children aged from 2 to 16 years of age have been found to have increased levels of the age-related gene DNA methylation (Wikenius et al. 2019). A particular concern of epigenetic research has therefore been with the effects of maternal nutrition and early-life stress effects. Yet the extent to which transmitted epigenetic information is modulated by the environment, and whether this process is adaptive across generations remains uncertain (Perez and Lehner 2019: 147). What has come to be termed 'classic epigenetics' are those studies that seek to identify the process of phenotypic change occurring during this period of early development or during early stages of the disease process. Here, alterations in chromatin structure that result in transcriptional activation (see Glossary) or repression are seen as indicators of epigenetic modification. This is because of the role of chromatin in DNA replication, gene expression, and differentiation (NHGRI 2019).

It is somewhat ironic that in the post-HGP era of pharmacogenomics and personal genomics (discussed in the previous chapter), generally seen as representing a breakthrough in the ability to identify and manage the DNA variants that caused disease traits within individual germlines, a different approach within molecular research has shifted the focus from the gene to the 'epi' that surrounds it; the reactivity of the genome to environmental signals (Pinel et al. 2018: 277). The bulk of epigenetic research on early development has been conducted using animal models, which 'are intended to serve as meaningful surrogates for the human situation' (Wastell and White 2017: 157). These experiments are conducted utilising the methodology of 'behavioural paradigms' that assess animal behaviour in response to artificial stimuli (both reward and stress inducements) and draw upon various assumptions about the processes of operant conditioned behaviour. These experimental methods typically involve shock treatments to rodents, including isolation, shaking, handling/non-handling, and maternal separation from pups to induce or to limit a stress response. The experimental focus is on the levels of the hormone corticosterone (see Glossary) produced in response to these stressors, measured by the levels of the hormone that bind to the glucocorticoid receptor (GR) in the hippocampus, a part of the brain associated with memory, learning, and emotions. Over time, this experimental work has constructed a body of evidence that points to the importance of maternal behaviour on GR expression, and hypothalamic pituitary adrenal (HPA—see Glossary) responses to stress in rat pups, mediated by alterations in chromatin structure, 'demonstrating a close relationship between elevated stress in early life and the appearance of behavioural disorders in later life' (Cunliffe 2015: 59 cited in Wastell and White 2017: 158).

The use of the maternal separation model in particular offers epigenetic research the opportunity to influence the experiences of care and to control for early-life adversity for the rat pups in early development. The stressors experienced by the pups in these experiments are linked to later behavioural changes, as well as potential epigenetic change such as hormone levels in the brain. The 'care' of these laboratory rodents is an important consideration when assessing the generalisability of this early development experimental research. 'Care' is essential for establishing research protocols that ensure a consistent experimental environmental experience is maintained. Such care protocols serve to stabilise particular facets of the experiment while preventing extraneous factors from influencing the final study results. That is, they serve to provide the basis for the reproducible measurement and analysis of the rodent brains and bodies. The care process enables lab-based researchers: 'to construct early-life adversity as a legible and influential experience that can have lasting impacts on behavioural health. These practices matter because they allow behavioural epigenetics to trace the molecular effects of particular experiences, elevating some forms of care as primary for health, while largely eclipsing others' (Lappé 2018: 700).

However, it is also important to be aware of the potential for over-determining the outcomes of an experimental process that manipulates the care environments of rodent pups. The artificial invocation of stress and/or care is designed to replicate the environmental stimuli of early-life adversity, any epigenetic modification in response to this environment is represented by a proxy measure, high or low HPA measurements. As Wastell and White have noted: '(T)he rat, as a sentient, cognitive creature attempting to deal with the challenges of its somewhat meagre life in the laboratory is utterly effaced by the reduction of parenting behaviour to the methylation of one gene in one brain structure… (T)he all-important imperative for the rat is long-term reproductive success, and there is nothing it can do to influence this (in the lab)' (2017: 165). These classic studies consistently draw conclusions about the correlation of 'environment' with neglectful or efficacious maternal behaviour and the subsequent outcomes for the adaptability of pups. Yet, for rats in the wild, it is their reproductive success that counts, not maternal caring performance in a laboratory experiment. The maternal bodies and behaviours of rodents that are measured in these experiments are necessarily 'staged as epigenetically meaningful in ways that preclude the consideration of the wider social and material environments in which mothers and children live' (Lloyd and Müller 2018: 676).

'Natural Experiments' and Human Epigenetic Research

A key concern for environmental epigenetics is just how far can the findings that are drawn from animal research be applied to human interactions and behaviour? In human societies, mothers are not isolated child-rearers, fathers, peer groups, kinship support structures, nurseries, and educational institutions all have a role in shaping the developmental potential of children. There are also clearly insurmountable ethical objections to conducting experiments with children, not least because such research would have no obvious direct benefits for these human subjects. These ethical concerns are certainly a key factor in the paucity of any large-scale research assessing epigenetic change in humans, even of the non-invasive sort: '(T)o the best of our knowledge, there have been no epigenome-wide association studies (EWAS) of DNA methylation changes in infants during the first year of life' (Wikenius et al. 2019).

However, what are known as 'natural experiments' (NE) or 'quasi-experimental events' do offer the potential for researchers to conduct, as near as possible, a form of unbiased comparison between similar population groups exposed or not, to a particular condition or event. The most well-known example of a quasi-experiment is the longitudinal research that has been conducted examining the impact of the Dutch Hunger Winter or 'Hongerwinter'. Towards the end of the Second World War in Europe, in the winter of 1944/45, the Western part of the Netherlands remained under Nazi occupation, while the Allied forces had recently liberated the Eastern part. The Nazi occupiers were therefore cut off Germany and from sufficient food supplies for the army, so they forcibly imposed a drastic regime of food rationing on the civilian population. The effects of this near starvation diet on the local population has subsequently been well documented so that there is more than sufficient longitudinal data available to enable researchers to assess any durable metabolic effects of rationing on children born in the occupied sector compared to babies born in the unoccupied sector (including a small sample of siblings separated across the two zones). This longitudinal data has provided an excellent resource for research carried out by Lumey et al. (2007) in a ground-breaking study that examined persistent epigenetic effects of a cohort exposed to this enforced famine at the time of their conception. The researchers were able to identify members of this cohort from the original records, then trace and interview them as adults age 43 (in 1998), then with further follow-up nearly a decade later. The findings were that for the small sample who were compared with their unexposed (to the starvation diet) same-sex siblings, an epigenetic 'tag', that is a small reduction in methylation levels of the maternally imprinted insulin growth factor IGF2 (an important factor in human growth and development), was found to have occurred. On this basis, Lumey et al.'s (2007) study has been claimed as 'the first to contribute empirical support for the hypothesis that early-life environmental conditions can cause epigenetic changes in humans that persist throughout life' (Heijmans et al. 2008: 17046).

However, Lumey et al.'s study of the effects of the Hongerwinter offered no clear epigenetic explanation for the methylation modification that was found in individuals more than six decades after their exposure to the starvation diet. Others have pointed out that 'although the mechanisms behind these relationships are unclear, an involvement of epigenetic dysregulation has been hypothesized' (Heijmans et al. 2008: 17049). Lumey et al.'s study also did not attempt to explain whether the reduction in IGF2 was dysfunctional or actually adaptive for these individuals (Wastell and White 2017: 182). A decade on from their original study, Lumey and his colleagues remain wedded to their original conclusions, arguing that their findings, together with the findings of similar epidemiological studies of the effect of famine, in the Ukraine in the 1930s, and during what was known as the 'Great Leap Forward' in China in 1959–1961: '(S)uggest that maternal nutrition during critical windows in gestation has a long-term impact on offspring's health and that exposure to large segments of the population can affect entire generations of people' (Skinner et al. 2019: 634). Yet these authors also acknowledge that there 'is a clear need for animal models to test this concept directly' (2019: 634). This conclusion is a de facto recognition of the tantalising but still complex and uncertain evidence for durable epigenetic effects in humans. Indeed, the small effects found in individuals who had experienced the Hongerwinter as babies may actually indicate that the experience of famine and hardship, which affected all groups within the population under Nazi occupation to a greater or less extent, appears to have had relatively little physical effect over the long term. This is likely to be due to the fact that while higher socioeconomic class status was found to have had little advantage in the extreme circumstances of wartime famine under enemy occupation, in the comparatively benign social conditions pertaining in psot-war contemporary Western Europe, social disadvantage does play a major role in inequalities in health outcome (Wastell and White 2017: 184).

Epigenetic Inheritance Research: The Transgenerational Imprinting of Social Behaviour?

The objective of this section is to critically engage with non-DNA sequence-based inheritance research. This research field within environmental epigenetics seeks to examine the ways in epigenetic modifications may be passed on across generations and as such represents one of epigenetics' most controversial lines of enquiry. Not least because of the ways in which research findings have been utilised in order to construct a biological explanation for transgenerational transmission of social inequalities and disruptive social behaviour. This is an approach that has informed public policy interventions within the USA but not yet the UK to any great extent.

The epistemological basis for conducting bioscience research into transgenerational effects has been summarised as follows: 'DNA is a reliable information transfer system because of the accuracy of DNA replication… (H) owever, eggs and sperm contain more than DNA, and it has become increasingly apparent in recent years that other molecules beyond the genome sequence can also transfer information between generations. Moreover, this information can be altered following change in the physiological and environmental conditions of previous generations' (Perez and Lehner 2019: 143). Within the epigenetic research field, 'only altered phenotypes occurring in the second (in the case of male transmission) or third (in the case of female transmission) generation after a trigger can truly be described as transgenerational inheritance. Effects spanning shorter timescales are described as parental or intergenerational. Nonetheless, many described intergenerational effects share mechanisms with transgenerational effects' (Perez and Lehner 2019: 143). The evidence for transgenerational epigenetic inheritance comes largely from rodent studies. Results from this experimental approach, described in detail above, indicate that pups produced from rodent mothers and fathers exposed to stressors produce similar 'depressive-like' behaviour across several rodent generations. This has led some epigeneticists to draw the firm conclusion that 'early stress alters DNA methylation in the male germline and that some of the alterations can be maintained and passed to the offspring' (Franklin et al. 2010: 413 cited in Wastell and White 2017: 173).

The focus of epigenetic inheritance research with humans has been with intergenerational obesity. Factors such as maternal body weight, nutrition before and during pregnancy, and the food intake of children in their early years have all been examined. To put it succinctly, the assumption underpinning this research is that 'its all about what we eat'. Many of these intergenerational studies utilise socioeconomic status (SES) as a key independent variable in their research design, in particular the reported association between higher body weight and poor nutrition in low SES mothers, both of which have been labelled as risk factors for childhood obesity. Given this focus, discussions of possible policy interventions often focus on educating mothers about how to eat better and lose weight before pregnancy (Müller et al. 2017: 1679). Interestingly, a Foresight Report (2007) commissioned by the UK government over a decade ago concluded that the significant increase that has occurred in rates of childhood obesity within just one to two generations reflects a complex set of social, cultural, and economic processes than cannot be explained by transmitted genetic effects. Social and structural factors would play at least as significant role as individual maternal behaviour in childhood obesity.

A particular criticism of transgenerational epigenetic studies is the implicit assumptions made about the cohorts that are being sampled, prior to any research being conducted. Adults and children are often chosen from pre-defined low-socioeconomic status groups known to be more likely to have experienced early trauma or that have poorer nutritional balance than the average in the UK or the USA. This sampling bias is problematic because the causes of epigenetic 'damage' then become inherently focused only on the more socially deprived and marginalised groups in society, reinforcing pre-existing stereotypes and stigma (Müller et al. 2017: 1680). Such conclusions often fail to take account of the limited social and economic opportunities for social mobility for these groups, and so unwittingly reinforce political ideologies that discuss poverty in terms of intergenerational inherited social deficits of various kinds rather than the effects of social structural inequality. Too often the attempt is made to politically expropriate and manipulate the findings of epigenetic research in order to reinforce long-standing prejudicial judgements about parenting styles and the role of mothers in society. But to give the last word to pair of epigeneticists, whose recent review of the evidence for transgenerational epigenetic inheritance concluded that:

> *Parental effects over a single generation can act via many mechanisms with phenotypic consequences. However, little evidence exists to date for multigenerational memory of physiological alterations following environmental changes, even though the potential for longer-lasting memories has been demonstrated (in animal models)...owing to the long duration of a single human generation, adaptive epigenetic inheritance seems unlikely over any generational timescale... Regardless of the species, parental experiences are more likely to predict environmental conditions than those of more distant ancestors.* (Perez and Lehner 2019: 155)

'Race' and Categories of Difference in Epigenetic Research

Historically, classifications of 'race'[1] have been used to identify some outward physical characteristic such as skin colour or hair texture or some reductionist quality of identifiable population groups. As such the label has been used to assert political, economic, and social power over minority groups, through the application of social, political, and institutional forms of discrimination. These structures of racism have had a long and disturbing history within many Western societies.

Within the natural sciences, taxonomies of racial difference were first established as early as the eighteenth century and subsequently played an important role in justifying slavery and the legitimacy of colonial rule in Africa, the Americas, South-east Asia, and elsewhere in the world. By the early decades of the twentieth century, a number of Mendelian geneticists were mobilising their research for the dubious purpose of identifying racial differences in intellectual ability and disease outcomes. Many of these scientists were committed eugenicists, a philosophy that asserted that debilitating mental and physical diseases were hereditary, and in some cases associated with 'inferior races'. It was on this basis that the eugenics movement proposed sterilisation or worse, in order to maintain the 'purity' or 'hygiene' of a society. This eugenicist outlook continued to have an influence within the work of

[1] The convention within sociology is to place the term 'race' within inverted commas to emphasis the fact that as a way of categorising individuals and population groups, it is not based on any scientifically valid distinctions. In this section that convention will be maintained in the context of its use within biomedical research studies. But where the term is utilised as a social construction and continues to have meaning in a particular social context, it will be used without the inverted commas.

some geneticists right up until the horrors of the Holocaust carried out by the Nazi's during the Second World War. Post-war biological research generally replaced the language of 'racial difference' with that of 'population group'. Yet inadvertently or not, this new category 'permitted ideas of race as biology to persist and sanitized the study of human genetic differences in an attempt to diffuse some of the post-World War II anxieties around race' (Rajagopalan et al. 2017: 353). Yet despite many attempts to establish a scientifically valid classification of 'race', the unambiguous outcome of the completion of the HGP sequencing programme in 2003 was that genetically discrete population categories do not exist.

Population groups cannot be scientifically differentiated by genotype. However, phenotypical characteristics including skin colour, body fat distribution, and disease susceptibility (crudely correlating with notions of 'race') are directly linked to the pre-history of human migration. This post-HGP understanding was acknowledged in the subsequent take-up of the concept of 'continental ancestry' in genetic research: '(I)t is more appropriate to specify that the genetic diversity we observe is due to continental ancestry rather than to "race"… (T)he current state of the evidence is that oft cited traits like sickle cell genotype and genes related to skin tone remain unique and rare examples of genetic differences that have persisted due to continental ancestry' (Rehkopf and Needham 2019: 54). The inference of continental ancestry is based on region-specific haplogroup diversity. This is group diversity defined by the sharing of a common ancestor with an SNP (see Glossary) mutation. The haplogroups most commonly studied are groups with Y-chromosome (Y-DNA) mutation passed along the patrilineal line and mitochondrial DNA (mtDNA) mutation passed down the matrilineal line.

Yet despite these developments in the understanding of genetic ancestry, 'race' as a population variable continues to make a frequent appearance in an extensive range of molecular and biomedical research papers, but rarely if ever defined. Reifying race as a biological category in explanations of patterns of disease susceptibility has a long and undignified history in biomedicine. Ethnic minorities (see Glossary) were often identified as problematically disease susceptible (before any understanding of modern genomics). In the late nineteenth century in New York and London, this form of stereotyping led on to the linking of outbreaks of TB with the Jewish population. Today, it is more likely to be Afro-American, Afro-Caribbean, or minorities from the Indian subcontinent that are highlighted in these 'disease-susceptibility' terms. Troy Duster has argued that in the post-genomic period '(A) significant wing of biological sciences has found an unusual and effective way around the problem of confronting the matter of race as a biological category. The strategy is not deal with the difficulties associated with defining "race" in a full-scale case-control design, but to "back it into" a clinical study that was never designed to test whether race plays any role' (Duster 2015: 12). While Barbara Prainsack (2016) has strongly asserted that because precision medicine relies on DNA markers of some aspects of phenotype, it rarely attributes ethnic minority differences in health outcome to environmental factors. As such, it inadvertently serves to act as a form of 'racialized medicine'. And within epigenetic research, 'race' as we shall see appears to have been 're-inscribed' as a biological category (Duster 2015: 2).

The vast majority of social scientists reject the conceptualisation of 'race' as a categorical or biological essentialist characteristic of a social group. But in general they would not seek to efface or eliminate it from social analysis. This is because it is seen as necessary to highlight the effects of socioeconomic and material disadvantage as they disproportionately impact on ethnic minority groups. Recognising the detrimental health and social impacts of a lifetime experience of being discriminated against on the grounds of race is to acknowledge the continuing existence of institutionalised and social forms of discriminatory practice. 'Race', as it continues to be used in some epigenetic research as a marker of human differentiation, is a social construction nothing more, but race used as the basis for an understanding of the persistence of social inequity is most certainly a real social phenomenon. So if it is reasonable to assume that the vast majority of genomic scientists are not covert or indeed overt racists, and that their training has inculcated in them the necessity of utilising a verifiable hypothetico-deductive scientific method, then the question arises as to what are the justifications for continuing to deploy the population category of 'race' in research?

One possible explanation is that 'race' has a practical predictive validity as a proxy measure, 'yielding reliable inferences or sound probabilistic reasoning in some specifically well-defined biomedical contexts without necessarily being a valid primary concept in human population genetics' (Maglo 2010: 362). Maglo goes on to argue that this is a justified use because 'instrumentalism only requires that race be an efficient, safe, and ethically defensible biomedical problem-solving device' (2010: 364). This argument may be formally correct on the strictly methodological point of using proxies to stand-in for less than well-understood variables of biological heterogeneity, but the argument for the ethical defensibility of using race on the grounds of scientific utility remains highly questionable. Other essentially social measures of population difference, such as gender, socioeconomic class, or self-identified ethnicity can be agreed upon in terms of their broad parameters, but the social construct of race carries with it an almost unbearable historical and cultural weight that cannot easily be put to one side. Genomic research does not and cannot exist in a social vacuum, so that the risks associated with this 're-inscription' of 'race' as a research category are ethically unsustainable.

We now turn to the question of the use of 'race' as a research category specifically within the field of environmental epigenetics. Epigenetics can reasonably be conceived as representing a paradigm shift in the field of genomics, 'a different style of reasoning…a radical rethinking of the ontology of the genome and even a dismissal of its role as the prime mover in biological processes' (Meloni 2017: 391). On this basis, Meloni sees epigenetics as representing a return to what he terms 'soft-heredity', an emphasis on the broader mechanisms of non-genetic inheritance. That is, human biology as shaped by environmental signals, rather than the internal transmission of nuclear DNA from one generation to another; the latter being termed 'hard-heredity'. But this paradigmatic shift has not led to the elimination of 'race' as a research category. Rather, epigenetic processes are positioned as a transgenerational pathway, where the social and environmental experiences of identified population groups are seen to travel through to the next generation and beyond. Unlike traditional genetics, post-genomic epigenetics does not seek to identify 'genes for' in order to explain differences in health outcomes between identified 'racial' groups. Rather, it seeks to identify the socio-historical conditions materialised over time in the bodies of these identified groups, mediated through processes of DNA methylation change.

On this basis, epigenetic research, especially in the USA, has sought to re-assess the significance of 'race' as a soft-heredity explanatory factor in the higher rates of disease experienced by African Americans (AAs). Examples of this trend would be the attempt to find an ancestral link from the experience of malnutrition and intense physical labour during the period of slavery in the nineteenth century to the high rates of low-birth-weight babies experienced by Afro-Americans in contemporary USA. The focus of Kuzawa and Sweet's study (2009) is not the intergenerational effects of slavery but the embodiment of the contemporary experience of racism and its negative effects on maternal biology. The stresses of racism in their research are seen to be transmitted in utero, which has had the effect of 'programming' the next generation for a higher risk of cardiovascular disease. But as Meloni (2017) has pointed out, it would be a mistake to equate the environmental epigenetics of Kuzawa and Sweet's research with, for example, a sociological approach that emphasises the social and material structural outcomes of institutional racism as having a direct impact in unequal health outcomes for ethnic minorities. The epigenetic molecular in utero conceptualisation of environment is of a very different epistemological order. In this 'epigenetic-developmentalist' model, '(T)he arrow is not only one-way from the social to the biological: the mechanism is bidirectional…the reciprocal interaction of social factors on biology and biological ones in shaping the milieus of future generations' (Meloni 2017: 397). This is an exposure to an epigenetic environment that confers physical disadvantage or advantage on future generations with apparently no possibilities for evasion.

Rehkopf and Needham (2019) have made a number of recommendations concerning the methodological conduct of epigenetic studies involving the use of 'race' or ethnicity as a research category in examining the impact of environmental factors on DNA methylation and subsequent health outcomes. They argue that if a study chooses to use the category 'race-ethnicity', then it should be clearly defined as a social, not a biological category. If examining the impact of environment on health outcomes, it is recommended that continental ancestry be used as an independent variable rather than race-ethnicity. The latter is a potential confounding factor in such research given that it incorporates and captures environmental-social difference. However, in practice many such epigenetic studies make little or no attempt to define their use of race as a category. Such studies are also rarely explicit as to their decision to use race or ethnicity rather than continental ancestry, and if both variables are used, they are often elided one with the other (Rehkopf and Needham 2019: 62).

The guidelines for the use of the category of 'race' in genetics research outlined by Rehkopf and Needham (2019) have its antecedents in immediate post-HGP concerns about the lack of clarity and consistency in the description of research populations and inadequate justification for their use in biomedical research. Journal editors, professional societies, and expert commentators have all offered a range of guidelines for the use and reporting of race and ethnicity in genetic research, these generally converge around four key points: (1) to define race and ethnicity in the context of a research study; (2) to explain how the terms or categories relate to the research hypothesis; (3) to describe how participants were assigned to the research populations; and (4) to describe the limitations of the study with respect to the populations to which the research findings can be generalised (Ali-Khan et al. 2011: 48). To assess the extent to which genetic scientists were following these guidelines in practice, Ali-Khan et al. conducted a systematic review of 170 population genetic research articles from high-impact journals published between 2008 and 2009, in order to assess how and when the categories 'race', 'ethnicity', and 'ancestry' were utilised. A comparative perspective was obtained by these authors in aligning their metrics with similar research from articles published in the period 2001–2004. The authors concluded:

> Our analysis indicates a marked improvement in compliance with some of the recommendations and guidelines for the use of race/ethnicity over time, while showing that important shortfalls still remain: no article using "race", "ethnicity" or "ancestry" defined or discussed the meaning of these concepts in context; a third of articles still do not provide a rationale for their use, with those using "ancestry" being the least likely to do so. Further, no article discussed potential socio-ethical implications of the reported research. (Ali-Khan et al. 2011: 58)

In order to see if there had been any marked shift in the adoption of definitional guidelines in the decade since Ali-Khan et al.'s paper was first published, a substantially pared down version of their review was carried out by IC (Table 7.1). This simple exercise sought to assess the extent to which relatively recent epigenetic research papers now provide comprehensive definitions of their population group variables. Five published papers that have appeared in the academic journal '*Epigenetics*', a highly cited publication within the field, were identified using the search terms 'race', 'racial', 'ethnicity', or 'ancestry' in the title of the paper. The five papers were assessed for the presence or absence of definitions, and whether or not racial or ethnic difference was attributed to DNA methylation (DNAm) level. The papers are cited in the number order appearing below:

1. Kumaraswamy et al. (2019) Race specific alterations in DNA methylation among middle-aged African American and Whites with metabolic syndrome.
2. Zhang, F et al. (2011) Significant differences in global genomic DNA methylation by gender and race/ethnicity in peripheral blood.
3. Song, M et al. (2015) Racial differences in genome-wide methylation profiling and gene expression in breast tissues from healthy women.
4. Daveney, J et al. (2014) Genome-wide differentially methylated genes in prostate cancer tissues from African American and Caucasian men.
5. Smith, J et al. (2017) Neighborhood characteristics influence DNA methylation of genes involved in stress response and inflammation: The Multi-Ethnic Study of Atherosclerosis.

In each of the five papers it was found that there was no attempt to define the central independent variable, race, and/or ethnicity. All these studies identify an environmental correlation between race and DNAm in relation to the aetiology of

Table 7.1 Epigenetic epidemiological studies in the Journal *Epigenetics*: Examining the impact of race and ethnicity on DNA methylation (DNAm)

Paper	Study objective	Definitions	Attribution of racial or ethnic differences
1	Examination of DNAm signatures measured across the genome associated with metabolic syndrome (a cluster of three or more cardiometabolic risk factors) using DNA from urban dwelling African American (AA) and White adult participants.	Race not defined	'DNAm differences might contribute to MetS risk among Whites and AAs since different genes were identified in AAs and Whites'. But noting that 'poverty status may have a race-specific role in regulating different molecular, cellular and biological processes'.
2	Explore and describe the relation of global leukocyte DNAm to ageing, demographics, and environmental factors (objective to identify epigenetic marker of cancer risk).	Race not defined. Ethnicity defined as Hispanic *or* non-Hispanic	'Significant differences found in global genomic DNAm by gender and race/ethnicity in a cancer-free population. The associations are unlikely to be mediated by body composition and other behavioral risk factors. The biological mechanisms underlying these differences warrant further investigation'.
3	Assess differences by race for genome-wide DNA methylation and gene expression in healthy women with no prior history of breast cancer.	Race defined by 'self-report': European American *or* African American	'Racial differences in DNAm exist among healthy women and that those methylation differences are correlated with gene expression at some levels, suggesting a contribution to racial disparities in breast cancer'.
4	Comparison of the genome-wide DNAm pattern in normal and prostate cancer tissue samples from AA and Caucasian men, correlated with gene expression in PCa samples from AA and Caucasian men.	Race not defined. Ethnicity not defined	'We have found that genome-wide methylation patterns differ by ethnic/racial groups, which suggest distinct differences in the etiology of PCa in AA vs. Caucasian'.
5	An examination of neighbourhood-level socioeconomic disadvantage and neighbourhood social environment as predictors of DNAm levels in eighteen genes related to stress reactivity and inflammation. The relationships evaluated in a large, multi-ethnic, population-based sample of US adults.	Ethnicity not defined, but sample divided into non-Hispanic White, Hispanic, AA	High socioeconomic disadvantage and worse social environment were primarily associated with increased methylation. Respondents living in a neighbourhood with greater socioeconomic disadvantage or a worse social environment were younger, were more likely to be female, Hispanic, or African American, and were more likely to have low socioeconomic status.

the particular disease being assessed. However, no causative biological explanation of why (or not) race correlates with differential health outcomes is provided in any of the papers. The elephant in the room, 'race' as a biological construct, is never directly addressed. The one interesting exception within this very selective sample is study number 5 (Smith et al. 2017). While not providing an explicit definition of 'ethnicity', the paper finds no significant correlation between this research category and DNAm associated with stress response, leading on to atherosclerosis. The most significant correlation is found to be between DNAm and living within a neighbourhood that is characterised by high socioeconomic disadvantage whatever the ethnic identity of the research subject.

A number of bioethicists have reflected upon the ways in which the social construction of 'race' continues to be utilised as a variable within mainstream epigenetics research. Perez-Rodriquez and de la Fuente (2017) have argued that its continued use justifies the shift to what they describe as a new 'post-racial' biomedicine. They argue that instead of looking for 'clustering similarities amongst groups of people sharing a physical resemblance', epigenetics should focus on the 'idiosyncratic genetic and environmental milieu' of individuals (not social groups) that leads on to such susceptibilities. However, there should be some wariness in rushing to embrace a 'post-racial' bioscience, given that social scientists continue to document the effects of racism as being real and enduring, despite the fallacy of biological race (Morrison and Granka 2017). Environmental epigenetics has an important role in contributing to the science of assessing the effects of social disadvantage on health outcomes but must be open to addressing its own methodological shortcomings in relation to race and ethnicity.

Constituting the 'Environment' in Epigenetics: Renegotiating the Biological-Social Boundary

In the second half of the twentieth century, there existed a notable complementarity between the social and the biomedical sciences, informed by epidemiological research, that population health outcomes were shaped by environmental determinants (alongside the influence of hereditary genetics). This association began to loosen towards the end of the century, as gene-centric 'hard-heredity' research came to dominate genomic science. However, in the post-genomic period, with the shift away from studying the human genome in isolation, questions about the ways in which our bodies are adapted by social, physical, and cultural environments are once again being posed.

Ostensibly, environmental epigenetics and its understanding of the plastic nature of genetic processes, 'falling within the parameters of the human life span' (Lappé and Landecker 2015: 153) and mediated by social experiences, has much in common with the Human Life Course approach influential in 'biopsychosocial' studies of health and ageing. That is, a common understanding of the dynamic 'embodiment' of social and environmental interactions. Meloni describes these developments as constituting 'the social turn' in biological sciences leading to a realignment or 'renegotiation' of the relationship between biology and sociology (Meloni 2014). To cite Nick Rose, 'at its best the turn to epigenetics marks a recognition of the inseparability of vitality and milieu which could give a crucial role for the social and human sciences in accounting for the shaping of vitality at the molecular level' (Rose 2013: 18). If this early optimism is subsequently matched by a rise in biosocial interdisciplinary research, then this would indeed mark a significant epistemological shift within the social sciences. The latter having a tendency to view the human body as a 'taken-for-granted' black box, in which 'human variation has been conventionally left for those concerned with the biological domain' (Palsson 2016: 102).

Yet looking at the potential for interdisciplinary social research a number of methodological challenges do arise. Pinel et al. (2018), in their review of the epigenetic environment literature, found that the understanding of the nature of interactions occurring between genes, epigenetic processes, and the environment is quite variable. These authors identified significantly different conceptions of the epigenetic environment in four sub-fields of epigenetics. The first field, gene expression research, is seen as making little reference to the environment other than the chromatin environment of cell programming. In contrast, the second field, molecular epigenetics concerned with the action of epigenetic change, focuses on the macro environment of social stressors, lifestyle factors, and toxic metals and chemicals. Clinical epigenetics as a third sub-field, which seeks to translate knowledge of epigenetic processes into clinical care, focuses on the extracellular microenvironment of cancer cells. While the fourth sub-field, epigenetic epidemiology concerned with disease risk in populations, is unsurprisingly focused on the social environment and lifestyle factors. Yet the authors ultimately conclude that it is possible to synthesis a consistent commonality in the ways in which the complex interactions between genes and the environment are operationalised in epigenetics: '(W)here the environment is framed as the active actor initiating the relationship, the genes are the invariant in the relationship, receiving signals, while epigenetics are framed as the mediators enabling communication between environment and genes' (Pinel et al. 2018: 289).

Then there is the question of the exposure to environments that confer physical disadvantage or possibly advantage for future generations, which in turn raises the issue of the possibility of biological plasticity acting as a check to the over-determination of inherited genetic influences. In this context, Lappé and Landecker (2015) have observed that although the epigenome is conceived of as plastic, the genome itself is generally seen to be fixed or static in the epigenetics literature. It is on this basis that the epigenetic process is best understood as a mutable mediator existing between a fixed genome and dynamic environment. The principle of plasticity should in principle apply over a lifetime of environmental exposures, with variations potentially being reversible. Nevertheless, within some fields of epigenetics, the plasticity of the epigenome appears to be strictly temporal. That is, as a process operating predominantly within the period of early child development, the 'critical window' of DNA methylation changes. This makes it difficult to establish points of epistemological commonality with social scientists and epidemiologists whose understanding is that the material environment is necessarily characterised by unpredictability and dynamic change.

Any cursory reading of social history would find many examples of rapid social and environmental change that have led on to significant population health improvement. One example would be the post-war state welfare policy interventions (primarily within Western European states) that brought about significant improvements in the health and educational outcomes of their national populations over the course of just one generation. The issue is that while most social scientists necessarily embrace unpredictability in the social world, the epistemology of the biomedical sciences is generally concerned to establish linear causality between natural world phenomenon, and therefore predictability, and epigenetics is no exception to this rule (Newton 2016: 125). These epistemological differences set considerable challenges for effective interdisciplinary working between the social and biological sciences, but this does not make collaboration impossible.

Chapter Summary—Key Points

- *Epigenetics emerged as a 'revolutionary' new framework for conceptualising the environment outside of the human body as 'bioactive'.*
- *The epigenome comprises all of the chemical compounds not part of the DNA sequence, but on or are attached to DNA regulating the expression of all the genes in the genome.*
- *Epigenetic modifications are understood to regulate gene expression by acting as gatekeepers, blocking or allowing access to a gene's chemical 'on/off' switches.*
- *Epigenetic processes are crucial to normal development and differentiation, but they also modified by environmental and social influences.*
- *Post-genomic epigenetics can be seen as representing a return to what can be termed 'soft-heredity', an emphasis on the broader mechanisms of non-genetic inheritance.*
- *Classic epigenetics studies are those that seek to identify the process of phenotypic change occurring during early development, usually in rodent models.*
- *In theory, the use of the maternal separation model offers the opportunity to influence the experiences of care and to control for early-life adversity in early development.*
- *A key concern for 'classic' epigenetics is just how far can the findings drawn from animal research be applied to human interactions and behaviour?*
- *'Natural experiments' or 'quasi-experimental events' offer the potential for epigenetics researchers to conduct a form of unbiased comparison between human subjects.*
- *Epigenetic research is drawn upon as a biological explanation for transgenerational transmission of poverty and social behaviour.*
- *Intergenerational epigenetic research can unwittingly serve to reinforce political ideologies that see poverty in terms of inherited social deficits of various kinds.*

- *Parental effects over a single generation act via many mechanisms with phenotypic consequences, little evidence exists for multigenerational physiological alterations.*
- *Classifications of 'race' have been used to identify some outward physical characteristic or some reductionist quality of identifiable population groups primariliy in order to assert power over these groups.*
- *Epigenetic studies rarely explicit about the decision to use race rather than continental ancestry as an independent variable.*
- *Post-HGP, the concept of race based on appearance is rejected as too crude for biology at the level of the human genome.*
- *In the 'epigenetic-developmentalist' model, the arrow is not one-way from the social to the biological: the mechanism is bidirectional.*
- *There are significantly different conceptions of the environmental 'epi' found in the four sub-fields of epigenetics.*
- *In the post-genomic era, there has been a shift away from studying the human genome in isolation; epigenetic questions are now posed about the ways in which our bodies are adapted by social, physical, and cultural environments.*

Bibliography

Ali-Khan, S., Krakowski, T., Tahir, R., & Daar, A. (2011). The Use of Race, Ethnicity and Ancestry in Human Genetic Research. *The HUGO (Human Genome Organisation) Journal, 5*, 47–63.

Cunliffe, V. (2015). Experience-Sensitive Epigenetic Mechanisms. Developmental Plasticity, and the Biological Embedding of Chronic Disease Risk. *Systems Biology and Medicine, 7*, 53–71.

Daveney, J., Wang, S., Furbert-Harris, P., Apprey, V., Ittman, M., & Wang, B.-D. (2014). Genome-Wide Differentially Methylated Genes in Prostate Cancer Tissues from African-American and Caucasian Men. *Epigenetics, 10*(4), 310–328.

Duster, T. (2015). A Post-Genomic Surprise. The Molecular Re-inscription of Race in Science, Law and Medicine. *The British Journal of Sociology, 66*(1), 1–27.

Foresight Report. (2007). *Tackling Obesities—Future Choices*. London: UK Government Office for Science.

Franklin, T., et al. (2010). Epigenetic Transmission of the Impact of Early Stress across Generations. *Biological Psychiatry, 68*, 408–415.

Handy, D., Castro, R., & Loscalazo, J. (2011). Epigenetic Modifications: Basic Mechanisms and Role in Cardiovascular Disease. *Circulation, 123*(19), 2145–2156.

Heijmans, B., Tobi, E., & Stein, E. (2008). Persistent Epigenetic Differences Associated with Prenatal Exposure to Famine in Humans. *Proceedings of the National Academy of Sciences, 105*, 17046–17049.

Kumaraswamy, N. C., et al. (2019). Race Specific Alterations in DNA Methylation Among Middle-Aged African American and Whites with Metabolic Syndrome. *Epigenetics, 14*. https://doi.org/10.1080/15592294.2019.1695340.

Kuzawa, C., & Sweet, E. (2009). Epigenetics and the Embodiment of Race: Developmental Origins of US Racial Disparities in Cardiovascular Health. *American Journal of Human Biology, 21*, 2–15.

Lappé, M. (2018). The Paradox of Care in Behavioral Epigenctics: Constructing Early Life Adversity in the Lab. *BioSocieties, 13*(4), 698–714.

Lappé, M., & Landecker, H. (2015). How the Genome Got a Life Span. *New Genetics and Society, 34*(2), 152–176.

Lloyd, S., & Müller, R. (2018). Situating the Biosocial: Empirical Engagements with Environmental Epigenetics from the Lab to the Clinic. *BioSocieties, 13*(4), 675–680.

Lumey, L., Stein, A., Kahn, H., Van der Pal de Bruin, K., Blauw, G., Zybert, P., & Susser, E. (2007). Cohort Profile: The Dutch Hunger Winter Families Study. *International Journal of Epidemiology, 36*(6), 1196–1204.

Maglo, K. (2010). Genomics and the Conundrum of Race: Some Epistemic and Ethical Considerations. *Perspectives in Biology and Medicine, 53*(3), 357–372.

Meloni, M. (2014). How Biology Became Social, and What It Means for Social Theory. *The Sociological Review, 62*(3), 593–614.

Meloni, M. (2017). Race in an Epigenetic Time: Thinking Biology in the Plural. *The British Journal of Sociology, 68*(3), 389–409.

Morrison, D., & Grzanka, P. (2017). Postracial Fantasies and the Reproduction of Scientific Racism. *Communication and Sociology*, 2.

Müller, R., Hanson, C., & 20 Other Authors. (2017). The Biosocial Genome? *EMBO Reports, 19*(10), 1677–1682.

National Human Genome Research Institute (NHGRI). (n.d.). Retrieved November 2019, from https://www.genome.gov/about-genomics/.

National Institutes of Health (NIH). (n.d.-b). *What Is Epigenetics?* Retrieved January 2020, from https://ghr.nlm.nih.gov/primer/howgeneswork/epigenome.

Newton, T. (2016). The Turn to Biology. In M. Meloni, S. Williams, & P. Martin (Eds.), *Biosocial Matters: Rethinking Sociology-Biology Relations in the Twenty-First Century* (pp. 117–133).

Palsson, G. (2016). Unstable Bodies: Biosocial Perspectives on Human Variation. In M. Meloni, S. Williams, & P. Martin (Eds.), *Biosocial Matters: Rethinking Sociology-Biology Relations in the Twenty-First Century* (pp. 100–116).

Perez, M., & Lehner, B. (2019). Intergenerational and Transgenerational Epigenetic Inheritance in Animals. *Nature Cell Biology, 21*(2), 143–159.

Perez-Rodriguez, J., & de la Fuente, A. (2017). Now is the Time for a Postracial Medicine: Biomedical Research, the National Institutes of Health, and the Perpetuation of Scientific Racism. *American Journal of Bioethics, 17*(9), 36–47.

Pinel, C., Prainsack, B., & McKevitt, C. (2018). Markers as Mediators: A Review and Synthesis of Epigenetics Literature. *Biosocieties, 13*(1), 276–303.

Prainsack, B. (2016). Through Thick and Thin: Data Rich Medicine in the Era of Personalisation. In J. Vollman (Ed.), *The Ethics of Personalised Medicine: Critical Perspectives* (pp. 161–175). London: Routledge.

Rajagopalan, R., Nelson, A., & Fujimura, J. (2017). Race and Science in the Twenty-First Century. In U. Felt, R. Fouché, C. Miller, & L. Smith-Doerr (Eds.), *The Handbook of Science and Technology Studies* (4th ed., pp. 349–378). London, England: MIT Press.

Rehkopf, D., & Needham, B. (2019). The Impact of Race and Ethnicity in the Social Epigenomic Regulation of Disease. *Nutritional Epigenetics, 14*, 51–65.

Rose, N. (2013). The Human Sciences in a Biological Age. *Theory, Culture, and Society, 30*(1), 3–34.

Skinner, N., Lumey, L., Fleming, T., Sapienza, C., Hoyo, C., Aronica, L., et al. (2019). RW-2018—Research Workshop: The Effect of Nutrition on Epigenetic Status, Growth, and Health. *Journal of Parenteral and Enteral Nutrition, 43*(5), 627–637.

Smith, J., Zhao, W., Wang, X., Ratliff, S., Mukherjee, B., Kardia, S., et al. (2017). Neighborhood Characteristics Influence DNA Methylation of Genes Involved in Stress Response and Inflammation: The Multi-Ethnic Study of Atherosclerosis. *Epigenetics, 12*(8), 662–673.

Song, M., et al. (2015). Racial Differences in Genome-Wide Methylation Profiling and Gene Expression in Breast Tissues from Healthy Women. *Epigenetics, 10*(12), 1177–1187.

Wastell, D., & White, S. (2017). *Blinded by Science: The Social Implications of Epigenetics and Neuroscience*. Bristol: Policy Press.

Wikenius, E., Moe, V., Smith, L., Heiervang, E., & Berglund, A. (2019). DNA Methylation Changes in Infants between 6 and 52 Weeks. *Scientific Reports, 9*, 17587.

Wright, J. (2013). Epigenetics: Reversible Tags. *Nature, 498*, S10–S11.

Zhang, F., et al. (2011). Significant Differences in Global Genomic DNA Methylation by Gender and Race/Ethnicity in Peripheral Blood. *Epigenetics, 6*(5), 623–629.

Gendering Biomedical Science

8

Abstract

This chapter has two main themes. The first primarily focuses on perceived biological sex differences that remain a potent source of bioscientific interest, particularly within the neurosciences. It goes onto explore some of the reasons why gendered relations of power continue to make their mark in science, manifested in the shaping of research questions, and the reinforcement of cultural and social gendered stereotypes. The second theme is gender inequity in science education and careers. The chapter explores the reasons why horizontal and vertical forms of gender segregation in STEM continue to exist within the UK and across Europe, and will assess the utility of the notion of the 'leaky pipeline', focusing largely on the current situation in the biomedical sciences.

Introduction

The major theme of this chapter is a discussion of why perceived biological sex differences remain such a potent source of bioscientific interest, particularly in the neurosciences. This is despite not because of the friability of the evidence supporting sex difference that has been marshalled over many years. Gendered relations of power continue to make their mark, shaping research questions and reinforcing social stereotypes about women's role in the biomedical science. A second theme explored in the chapter is an assessment of the social and cultural factors that continue to perpetuate gender inequity in science education and careers, focusing largely on the current situation in the biomedical sciences.

From an STS perspective, gendering in science would be examined in terms of the ways in which the male norm becomes 'inscribed' within the design and structure of technologies of science (Fishman et al. 2017). While the contribution of the STS studies is acknowledged in this chapter, the discussion also draws on a wider

I. Crinson, *The Biomedical Sciences in Society*,
https://doi.org/10.1007/978-981-15-9523-3_8

range of interdisciplinary literature. This research is characterised by its engagement with the scientific, cultural, and historical contingencies associated with the structuring of gender bias in biomedical science practice. Before commencing a review of these themes it is necessary to clearly demarcate the analytical differences that exist between the concept of 'gender' and that of 'sex'. This task is necessary given that all too often, both terms continue to be used interchangeably in published biomedical science research papers.

'Female' and 'male' are biological categories that reference sex chromosomal differences. Humans and all mammals have two sex chromosomes, the X and the Y. Females have two X chromosomes in their cells, while males have both an X and a Y chromosome. However, the term 'sex' is not used solely to describe the biological reproductive features of human bodies, it is also used as the basis for mapping features of difference that are essentially social characteristics. In order to avoid this conflation and to distinguish between the biological fact of 'sex', and the social and cultural construction of masculine and feminine characteristics, social scientists utilise the term 'gender' to describe the latter. The distinction is not a question of semantics as is sometimes implied. Sex and gender are distinct analytical categories, and this is particularly pertinent given the existence of individuals who are not easily categorised by their external (biological) genitalia and by others who feel their anatomical body is out of line with their subjective sense of being masculine or feminine. Finally, it should be noted that the use of the term 'sex difference' within this textbook is strictly on the basis that many of the biomedical research studies that are described i have themselves divided-up participants on the basis of whether they are biologically female or male individuals. The term 'gender' is reserved for the analysis of socialisation and identity issues that are analytically pertinent when discussing career opportunities and segregation in biomedical science careers.

The 'Female Brain' and Other Gender Myths

Gender-based social stereotypes do not derive from 'natural' differences existing between men and women; they are rooted in the history of patriarchal relations of power. Patriarchy is usually defined as 'a system of social structures and practices in which men dominate, oppress and exploit women' (Walby 1989, 214). Patriarchy has a material reality in shaping the processes of socialisation that can result in distinct differences between young men and women in terms of the perceptions, expectations, and choices they make in relation to their education and careers. Gender-based social assumptions also take-on a material form when uncritically incorporated within research science.

In the late nineteenth century and early to mid-twentieth century, biological assertions of innate difference between the 'sexes' were a common currency in psychology and neurological science. Initially focused on brain size (no difference when corrected for overall body mass), then intelligence (no difference in overall IQ scores), this form of scientism was rooted in unchallenged social assumptions and served to justify the exclusion of women from higher education and the professions (other than the so-called caring professions of teaching and nursing) until when into the twentieth century.

Nevertheless, the attempt to provide a biological explanation for what are socialised gender identities continues to remain a topic of almost obsessive interest in some fields of biomedical science to this day. Complementary to this history of essentialising gender difference can be found an unconscious bias in bioscience that has long presented the male body as the biological template for the human species. *Portia Ltd* is a company that specialises in the design and implementation of evidence-based strategies for advancing quality of research and innovation through gender. In the evidence that this organisation presented to a House of Commons Select Committee investigation into women's career opportunities in science, it was stated that: '(T)he historical absence of women in research—as participants, as subjects, and as beneficiaries, has resulted in science having more evidence for men than for women, and in the 'male' being accepted as the norm in study design, and in the application and communication of research' (HoC 2014, 9).

The evidence that was presented to this Select Committee cites four examples of the 'male norm' in science. The first example was the lack of female crash dummies despite the obvious differences in male and female anatomy. Car accident injury statistics from the mid-1960s onwards show that on average females are exposed to double the risk of sustaining whiplash injuries than males. Female crash test dummies do exist, but they are not mandated to be used in most safety tests. In the European Union, five regulatory tests are used to assess adult occupant safety in the event of a crash. And, although regulatory tests worldwide display several local differences, they are all broadly similar to the European tests, which exclusively use the 50th percentile male to represent the whole adult population (Linder and Svedberg 2019, 158). The second example presented to the committee concerned the scientific understanding of physical pain, which was said to be based on the animal model of the male rat. This fact has only belatedly been acknowledged in the neurosciences, as the following quotation taken from a paper published in *Nature* argues: 'Most basic pain experiments test young adult, male Sprague Dawley rats, implicitly assuming that the biology that underlies pain processing and modulation in this organism is relevant to that of a chronic pain patient. Aside from possible species differences, this assumption is clearly belied by epidemiological evidence: the typical chronic-pain patient is middle-aged and female' (Mogil 2009, 285). The third example that was cited focused on how radiation dosage exposure calculations were made. These were said to continue to be based on the absorption model of a middle-aged man. The final example presented to the Select Committee was that up until relatively recently, the majority of images in anatomy and physiology textbooks (aside from the chapters on reproduction!) were of male bodies.

However popular the eponymous metaphor 'Men are from Mars, Women are from Venus' might be in everyday cultural exchanges, such simplistic forms of reductionism should have no place in rational scientific research, yet they continue to do so. In the last few years, an increasing number of (not exclusively) women scientists have set themselves the very necessary task of unravelling the assumptions of a 'gender-essentialist' neuroscience. Three of the more prominent examples of this critical literature that have been published over the past decade are Cordelia Fine's '*Delusions of Gender: The Real science behind Sex Differences*' (2010), Daphna Joel et al.'s '*Sex beyond the Genitalia: The Human Brain Mosaic*' (2015), and Gina Rippon's '*The Gendered Brain*' (2019). A selection of examples are drawn from each of these books in order to illustrate the ways in biological research science continues to essentialise gender difference.

Cordelia Fine published her 'Delusions of Gender' a decade ago to general critical acclaim. This book is not a peer-reviewed academic text as such, but it is a well-researched (the bibliography runs to thirty pages) broadside against what Fine terms 'neurosexism', the flawed notion that the male and female brain differs in ways that matter. As the review of this book in the *Guardian* newspaper makes clear, 'If we think we have left behind the cliché "Men think and women feel", Fine persuades us to think again. Newer, shinier versions take hold every year…(Fine) draws together research that shows people who pride themselves on their lack of bias persist in making stereotypical associations just below the threshold of consciousness' (Apter 2010). Fine's critique of neurosexism runs alongside a discussion of the reductionist gaze often found in the application of fMRI technology (discussed in Chap. 4 of this book).

A particular target of Fine's criticism is the oft-quoted book written by the psychologist Simon Baron-Cohen, forthrightly entitled '*The Essential Difference*' (2003). Baron-Cohen's book is constructed around the 'essential' position that 'the female brain is predominantly hardwired for empathy (while) the male brain is predominantly hardwired for understanding and building systems'. Baron-Cohen's conclusions about female empathy rest on the application of his own EQ (Empathy Quotient) questionnaire, and his research conclusions that people who score higher on the 'empathy scale' have 'female' brains, while the opposite result indicates a 'male' brain. Baron-Cohen's EQ questionnaire asked people to rank their own levels of sensitivity, and it is therefore not difficult to think of a plausible range of social causative hypotheses accounting for why women score relatively higher than men (Fine 2010;17). These factors might include the view that as children develop they are inculcated or socialised into society's expectations concerning normative gender roles, and subsequently, they act in accordance with these social expectations. Women are expected to be empathetic; therefore, if a women is asked a question about her levels of empathy in a questionnaire, she is more likely than not to score herself highly in this regard, with men having the opposite reaction. Fine is also highly critical of research that seeks to explain a propensity for empathy and caring by reference to the apparent difference of in utero levels of the hormone testosterone in mammalian male and female foetuses. Known as 'brain organisation theory', the evidence such as it is, is based on animal models and the experimental manipulation of hormonal environments of young rodent pups during the early critical periods of brain development. Extrapolating results from animal experiments in neuroendocrinology to draw hypothetical conclusions about the influence of testosterone on the much more complex brains of humans should be hedged with extreme caution. Nevertheless these considerations have not held back some scientists from discussing the uniqueness of the 'female' brain and ignoring the cultural processes of gender socialisation.

In her critique, Fine also points to the importance of the '5% rule' in which sex *differences* but not gender *similarities*, are reported in academic papers. This 'rule' relates to the *p* test of statistical probability where the difference between two groups or events could have occurred by chance. A rule of thumb is that any observed difference is seen as statistically significant if the probability that it could have occurred by chance is 1:20, or less. As Fine points out, the possibility of getting significant results by chance is a problem in any area of research, but is particularly the case for sex difference research. She demonstrates this point with the following example: A neuroscientist might be interested in what parts of the brain are involved in mind reading, and so brain scans fifteen participants asking them to guess the emotion of people in a selection of photographs presented to them. Since there are both men and women in the group, a quick check is run to ensure that the two groups' brains respond in the same way. They do. What does the scientist do next? Most likely, they publish their results without mentioning gender, except to note the numbers of males and females in the study. That neuroscientist is also seen as unlikely to publish their findings with the title, 'No Sex Difference's in Neural Circuitry involved in Understanding Others Minds'. This is reasonable given that this scientist was not overtly looking for gender difference. But even if men and women respond the same way overall on a given task, 5% of all studies will throw up a 'significant' difference between the sexes, purely by chance. As it is more interesting to find a difference than to find no difference, those 95% of studies that fail to observe significant sex differences and do not mention gender as a factor are less likely to be published. Whereas the 5% of studies that do observe a difference, even by chance, are more likely to be published. It is this one-in-twenty study that will then be cited in the media and elsewhere as evidence supporting the stereotype of gender difference, not the nineteen unpublished studies that found no difference (Fine 2010;134). An additional factor here is the 'seductive allure' of fMRI-based studies, particularly if they can be colour-coded to link some brain structure to 'sex difference' (this issue of 'allure' of brain imaging was discussed in Chap. 4).

Daphna Joel et al.'s (2015) study of sex difference in human brains sets out to challenge the sexually dimorphic (see Glossary) approach to neuroscience research that sustains the idea of the existence of the 'female' and 'male' brain. This approach is reflected in perceived sex differences in behaviour, cognition, personality, attitudes, and other characteristics that social scientists would generally see as being gendered. The authors make the logical conjecture that such a distinction would only be possible if sex differences in brain features were highly dimorphic, that is, with little or no overlap between the form of these features in males and in females. And additionally that those dimorphic brains if they existed would be internally consistent in terms of the 'maleness' or 'femaleness' in all of their neurological elements. Such an alignment it is argued would be predicted by the view of sexual differentiation, as being under the sole influence of testosterone levels in utero (Joel et al. 2015, 154568).

Joel et al.'s research sets out to test this internal consistency hypothesis. They analysed the MRI scans of more than 1400 human brains drawn from four datasets. In each dataset, the researchers focused on the brain regions that were said (in the dimorphic brain literature) to demonstrate the largest sex differences, that is, the least overlap between females and males. They found from their analysis of the scanning databases that there were in fact considerable overlap in these regions between the distributions of females and males, which made a division into two distinct forms impossible. Therefore, and to quote the paper, 'we tested whether individuals would be consistently at one end of the "femaleness-maleness" continuum across brain regions or show "substantial variability", being at the one end of the "femaleness-maleness" continuum on some regions and at the other end on other regions. We found that regardless of sample, type of MRI, and method of analysis, substantial variability is much more prevalent than internal consistency' (Joel et al. 2015, 15469). In the concluding discussion, and consistent with the findings of several other cited sources, the authors stated that:

> *Our analysis of the structure of the human brain, which included most regions of gray and white matter, as well as measures of connectivity, revealed many non-dimorphic group-level sex/gender differences in brain structure. There was extensive overlap of the distributions of females and males for all brain regions and connections assessed, irrespective of the type of sample, measure, or analysis (including analysis of absolute brain volumes). This extensive overlap undermines any attempt to distinguish between a "male" and a "female" form for specific brain features. Rather, the forms that are evident in most females are also the ones evident in most males. It is therefore more appropriate and informative to refer to measures of the brain in quantitative ways rather than in qualitative ways.* (Joel et al. 2015, 15471)

The publication of Daphna Joel and her team's study had a significant impact on the subsequent reception of sex difference research and served to undermine the myth of the female brain. While there were a number of subsequent attempts to challenge the study's methodology, the basic message that the brain is essentially a unique plastic pattern of features has not since been emphatically disputed. As the study concluded, 'most humans possess a mosaic of personality traits, attitudes, interests, and behaviors, some more common in males compared with females, others more common in females compared with males, and still others common in both females and males' (Joel et al. 2015, 15472).

Gina Rippon's (2019) book is a more recent addition to the sex difference debunking literature. This text, like that of Cordelia Fine's, is aimed at a 'popular science' audience, and also like Fine's work, it is packed with peer-reviewed references to back-up the substantive critique. Before embarking on her analysis of brain myths, Rippon discusses the ways in which women's, but rarely men's, behaviour has historically been biologised. Not just in terms of brain difference myths, but also in relation to hormonal change during the natural process of menstruation. The notion of premenstrual syndrome (PMS) first emerged in the 1930s and sought to link the new scientific understanding of the changes in hormonal levels prior to menstruation with apparently labile or irrational behaviour ('premenstrual tension'). By the 1960s, the notion of PMS linking biological and behaviour changes in women had entered popular culture. Rippon cites the example of NASA barring women from participating in the US space programme at this time, on the grounds that it would be inadvisable to have such 'temperamental psycho-physiologic humans' on board a spacecraft (Ryan et al. 2009 cited in Rippon 2019, 29). Rippon goes on to assert that the concept of PMS has now become so well established that it has become a self-fulfilling explanation for many women for the tensions and reactions they may be experiencing that could just as well have been attributed to other social and relational factors. Current science is of the consensual view that rather than negative irrational behaviour being associated with the ovulatory and post-ovulatory phases of the menstrual cycle, this period is associated with improved cognitive and affective processing. While some women certainly do have negative physical and emotional issues linked to hormonal fluctuations, the stereotype of PMS has become the universal myth associated with the experience of all premenstrual women (Rippon 2019, 31).

As we have seen in the discussion of 'brain organisation theory' above, the notion of PMS also makes the assumption that males and females are fundamentally different because the hormonal chemicals that determine their reproductive functioning also determine distinct functional and behavioural attributes. The retort offered to this assertion is that 'brains unlike genitals, are plastic' (Jordan-Young 2011, 289—cited in Rippon 2019, 38). The reductionist biological assumption that human development is context free, that outcomes are inevitable regardless of social expectations or cultural influences, is just poor science in the post-genomic era. Baron-Cohen's notion of 'male' brains orientated to 'things' and 'female' brains to people or empathy serves only to reinforce a powerful myth, one that plays to gendered cultural stereotypes. The biologisation of gender difference then essentially becomes an 'endorsement of the status quo; women as not suited to science work' (Rippon 2019, 241).

Another area of biologised sex difference research that has generated a lot of heat but little light over the years is the issue of sex differences in spatial cognition. Spatial cognition is conceived of as a general capacity, a 'fixed brain skill' which ranges from the ability to successfully move around the local environment, to reading maps and plans, to the ability to mentally manipulate abstract objects. When neuroscientists seek to measure spatial cognition, or 'visual-spatial processing', they generally are assessing performance on what is known as a mental rotation task (MRT). This basically involves the ability to mentally rotate a 3D figure so that it matches a second version. Research seems to suggest that boys are better than girls, but with considerable overlap, and that this just may have something to do with testosterone levels in utero. But further research has also demonstrated that sex differences in MRT performance might not be as stable as the essentialist view would suggest. While the neuro-imaging evidence is that men have greater surface area in the left parietal cortex, all this does is raise again the question of whether size actually matters in relation to brain structure? It should also be noted that MRT performance can improve with training to the point where sex differences disappear. This points to the importance of plasticity in brain functionality, not as a capacity somehow fixed by in utero sex differences. It would appear to be that 'fundamental sex difference is not so fundamental after all' (Rippon 2019, 274).

'Leaky Pipelines' and Gendered Roles in Biomedical Science Careers

When we look at science careers in the UK in the third decade of the twenty-first century, we continue to find that women remain significantly under-represented in most core STEM (science, technology, engineering, and mathematics) careers, *constituting just some* 24% of the workforce in 2019 (WISE 2019). This believe it or not represents an improvement on the 18% participation figure of a decade ago, but still nowhere near meeting the very modest goal of 30% of core STEM roles being filled by women by the year 2030, set by the Women in Science, Engineering and Technology (WISE) lobby group. The UK is by no means an outlier in terms of the marked gendered segregation found among its science workforce. Across most high-income countries, the same patterns of gender segregation are evident.

Attention at this point should be drawn to the analytical distinction that is drawn between two distinct types of gender segregation in the labour market. 'Horizontal segregation' is broadly defined as the relative concentration of men and women in different kinds of jobs, 'where the under-representation or over-representation of a given group in occupations or sectors is not ordered by any criterion' (EC 2009b). While 'vertical segregation' denotes the situation where for a particular gender opportunities for career progression within a given employment sector are more or less limited. This can contribute to a range of gender-related inequalities such as a gap in pay for similar work, and under-representation in senior and management positions in the workplace.

One starting point in identifying the origins of gender segregation in science careers is to look at gender differences in participation and performance in maths and the science subjects throughout school education. In the UK in 2009, just 16.7% of young women were entered for at least two science or maths A-levels compared to 28.5% of young men. A decade later in 2019, this number had increased to 22.1%, but over the same period, there was a similar proportional increase among in male students up to 34.7% undertaking two or more science or maths A-levels. Overall the gender balance in STEM subject uptake at A-level has remained broadly fixed, with the notable exception of biology. Looking in detail at the gender mix of science subjects, around three times as many males as females were undertaking physics in 2019, but nearly twice as many females as males were taking biology (Department of Education 2019). This picture is replicated in higher education in the UK, where the proportion of men studying natural science subjects remains considerably higher than the proportion of women, but there is a considerable variation between the fields of science. The Higher Education and Skills Agency (HESA) statistics showed that one of the fastest growing areas is 'subjects allied to medicine', where women students now constitute 80% of the total. In the biological sciences, women constitute the majority (65%) of students, as they also do in medicine and dentistry (60%).

The picture in physics, maths, engineering, and computer studies is reversed, with women constituting the minority of students—just 18% in engineering (HESA 2019).

Looking at post-university careers in the biomedical science employment sector in the UK, outside of academic and research roles in universities and research institutes (discussed below), there are three types of employer, Big Pharma, medical technology companies, and the expanding digital health sector. Generally speaking, horizontal segregation is not as marked in these sectors as in other core STEM sectors of employment. For example in engineering, women occupy just 10.3% of professional roles, and in Information Technology just 16.4% of professional roles. Nevertheless, the biomedical employment sector continues to be marked by significant pay gaps and limited opportunities for promotion to senior positions for women, that is, significant levels of vertical segregation exist. According to an analysis conducted by the science journal *Nature* that draws on gender pay statistics first released in the UK in 2017, pharmaceutical companies, medical technology, and other bioscience-focused organisations maintain a pay gap between men and women that is 50% greater than the national average. This equates to a median pay difference of +15% in favour of men. The pharmaceutical industry in particular has large variations in the pay. MSD, the UK subsidiary of Merck, had a +7% pay gap in favour of women, while GlaxoSmithKline (GSK) reported small differences in pay that favoured men. Pfizer and AstraZeneca, on the other hand, had gender pay gaps of 18% and 13%, respectively, in favour of men. This situation was seen to reflect the proportionately small numbers of women in senior roles across the sector (*Nature*: 'Science's vast gender pay gap revealed in UK wage data'—10 April 2018).

Examining the 2019 statistics for UK universities, of the 39,000 academic posts in the 'cost-centre' designated as 'medicine, dentistry and health', we find over 60% of academic posts held by women. But in the natural sciences, formally designated as 'biological, mathematical and physical sciences', women held just 33% of the 20,000 posts. Men hold the majority of academic posts overall in natural science, although the gender split is closest in the biosciences, where women hold 46% of the 14,500 posts (HESA 2019). In terms of vertical segregation, UK universities in 2019 reported a median gender pay gap of 13.7% in favour of men, with medical schools reporting an even larger gender pay gap in favour of men than the majority of HE institutions (PSA 2019). Outside of the UK, the picture of gender segregation is not much brighter. The European Commission have published what are known as the 'She figures' every three years, beginning in 2003. This data enables progress in meeting the goal of gender equality in science and technology occupations across the European Union to be monitored, providing an overview of the performance of individual member states on a wide range of indicators. The 2018 report (European Commission 2019) showed that only one-third of science researchers in the EU's twenty-eight member states are women, a situation which is unchanged since the previous report in 2015. Women across the EU were found to be more likely to graduate in natural science studies than men, and these numbers have grown over the period 2013–2016, but women were less likely than men to go on to doctoral-level study and pursue professional careers in these fields.

So what explanations are offered for these gender differences in education and science careers? One of the more common explanations deploys the metaphor of the 'leaky pipeline' to describe the path from post-16 education on to senior positions in science institutions and corporations. The 'leaky pipeline' represents the disproportional loss of women at each stage of the education and career pathway, but the model does not present this process as an explicit 'filtering out' of women from the STEM stream. As a descriptive schematic the leaky pipeline metaphor has its uses but it is not an explanation of gender segregation in science careers. For that we have to look to a range of sociological research that focuses on the impact of internalised gendered identities and the ways in which these can become self-fulfilling prophecies in terms of a choice of career. The educational interest and perseverance of young people in STEM subjects is seen as strongly tied to the differential processes of socialisation experienced by girls and boys both inside and outside school and home settings. Sociological research involving classroom observations of teacher and pupil interactions have indicated that science and maths teachers, regardless of their gender, tend to provide boys with more support, opportunities, and praise than girls. This finding reflects the continuing strength of social and cultural stereotypes that question young women's 'innate ability' in science and mathematics. These stereotypes implicitly tie in with the 'scientistic' belief in the existence of a sexually diamorphic human brain (discussed above).

Gendered social identities and differential normative assumptions concerning educational and career achievement can promote a sense of inferiority amongst young women leading to low expectations in relation to academic study and career choices (Hughes 2011, 549). Looking for the presence or absence of female role models 'is one way of looking at the environment that girls and women encounter as they learn science, rather than blaming female students for their situation' (Blickenstaff 2005, 376). Educational research points to the existence of gender differences in expressed attitudes, with young women typically expressing discomfort with the physical sciences, but less so the life sciences including biology (Ryan 2012). If career choices are closely tied to gender stereotypes, then this explains in part why many young women are attracted to those employment fields perceived as offering capacity to care for others, to improve the quality of life for others, and to have a social relevance that makes a positive difference in the world. A career in the biomedical sciences may be seen as fulfilling many of these concerns for young women (Kyte and Riegle-Crumb 2017, 13).

There is also the evidence that those women who are able to go on and become successful scientists frequently have had to make great personal sacrifices to compete on a level playing field with their male colleagues. As Ceci and Williams point out, 'the tenure structure in academe demands that women having children make their greatest intellectual contributions contemporaneously with their greatest physical and emotional achievements, a feat not expected of men' (2011, 3161). Women scientists often face a particular struggle in attempting to achieve a good work-home balance, between the demands of having a family and the time requirements necessary to pursue a successful research career. This situation is not of course unique to women scientists, but there continues to remain a strong gender bias in the 'domestic division of labour' (see Glossary) even within comparatively wealthy countries. Men typically still do not have to face the same level of push-pull constraints of family and work that women often do. This wider social structural context can be exacerbated by blinkered employment practices. For example, in the university sector it continues to be the case that there is a broad disinclination for employers to instigate effective 'family-friendly' policies that would enable staff (both men and women) to stop their 'tenure clocks'. A common experience for many academics after childbirth is that of having to return to their research roles on a part-time basis, because of the expense, availability, and restricted opening hours of pre-school childcare provision in the UK.

A firm commitment by employers, not just to the letter of a policy or procedure but to the spirit of gender equality, would provide both women and men with the flexibility to make the choice about whether to have children without detrimental consequences to their long-term careers. Gender segregation and inequality in science careers represent a loss of valuable human potential that could otherwise be usefully employed addressing many of the scientific and technological challenges we face in seeking to improve human health and well-being. Here both the biomedical and social sciences have an important role in challenging unscientific and gender-biased assumptions and to address the continuing exclusion of those that do not fit the model of the normative male.

Chapter Summary—Key Points

- *Necessary to distinguish between biological 'sex' and the cultural characteristics associated with being 'masculine' or 'feminine' represented by the concept of 'gender'.*
- *The term 'sex difference' is used when individuals are divided on the basis of being biologically female or male. The term 'gender' is reserved for the analysis of socialisation.*
- *Complementary to the essentialising of gender difference can be found a history of bias in bioscience that has presented the male body as the template for the human species.*
- *'Neurosexism' is the notion that male and female brains differ in ways that matter—a sexually dimorphic view of human behaviour, cognition, and perception.*
- *The reductionist notion of 'male' brains orientated to 'things' and 'female' brains to empathy, this remains a powerful myth that plays to many cultural stereotypes.*
- *Patriarchal power relations within the labour market, education system, and other civic institutions establish a 'gender order' marked by segregation and inequity.*
- ***Horizontal segregation** is defined as the relative concentration of men and women in different kinds of jobs.*
- *Vertical segregation denotes the situation whereby opportunities for career progression for a particular gender within a sector are more or less limited.*
- *Those young women who perceive the natural sciences as socially relevant are more likely to pursue careers in this field, a normative consideration not shared by young men.*

- *The history of interventions to address gender inequality in science education and careers, including gender mainstreaming, has been somewhat mixed in the UK.*

Bibliography

Apter, T. (2010). Delusions of Gender: The Real Science Behind Sex Differences by Cordelia Fine—Review. *Guardian*, 11 October 2010.

Blickenstaff, J. (2005). Women and Science Careers: Leaky Pipeline or Gender Filter? *Gender and Education, 17*(4), 369–386.

Ceci, S., & Williams, W. (2011). Understanding the current causes of women's underrepresentation in science. *PNAS, 108*(8), 3157–3162.

Department of Education. (2019). *A-Level and Other 16–18 Results: 2018–19 (Revised): Maths and Science Tables.* Retrieved from https://www.gov.uk/government/organisations/department-for-education.

European Commission. (2019). *She Figures 2018*. Brussels: European Commission.

Fine, C. (2010). *Delusions of Gender*. London: Iconbooks.

Fishman, J., Mamo, L., & Grzanka, P. (2017). Sex, Gender and sexuality in Biomedicine. In U. Felt, R. Fouché, C. Miller, & L. Smith-Doerr (Eds.), *The Handbook of Science and Technology Studies* (4th ed., pp. 379–406). London, England: MIT Press.

Higher Education Statistics Agency. (2019). *What Do HE Students Study?* Retrieved from https://www.hesa.ac.uk/data-and-analysis/students/what-study.

House of Commons Science and Technology Select Committee. (2014). Women in Scientific Careers—Sixth Report of Session 2013–14. HC 701. http://www.publications.parliament.uk/pa/cm201314/cmselect/cmsctech/701/701.pdf.

Hughes, R. (2011). Are the Predictors of Women's Persistence in STEM Painting the Full Picture? *Gender, Science and Technology, 3*(3), 547–570.

Joel, D., et al. (2015). Sex Beyond the Genitalia: The Human Brain mosaic. *Proceedings of the National Academy of Sciences of the USA, 112*(50), 15468–15473.

Jordan-Young, R. (2011). *Brainstorm: The Flaws in the Science of Sex Difference*. Cambridge, MA: Harvard University Press.

Kyte, S., & Riegle-Crumb, C. (2017). Perceptions of the Social Relevance of Science: Exploring the Implications for Gendered Patterns in Expectations of Majoring in STEM Fields. *Social Sciences, 6*(19), 1–13.

Linder, A., & Svedberg, W. (2019). Review of Average Sized Male and Female Occupant Models in European Regulatory Safety Assessment Tests and European Laws: Gaps and Bridging Suggestions. *Accident Analysis and Prevention, 127*, 156–162.

Mogil, J. (2009). Animal Models of Pain: Progress and Challenges. *Nature Reviews—Neuroscience, 10*, 283–294.

Political Science Association—PSA. (2019). Why Do UK Universities Have Such Large Gender Pay Gaps? Retrieved December 2019, from https://www.psa.ac.uk/psa/news/why-do-uk-universities-have-such-large-gender-pay-gaps.

Rippon, G. (2019). *The Gendered Brain*. London: The Bodley Head.

Ryan, L. (2012). 'You Must Be Very Intelligent…?': Gender and Science Subject Uptake. *International Journal of Gender, Science and Technology, 4*(2), 167–190.

Ryan, K., Loeppky, J., & Kilgore, D. (2009). A Forgotten Moment in Physiology: The Lovelace Women in Space Programme. *Advances in Physiology Education, 33*(3), 157–164.

Walby, S. (1989). Theorising Patriarchy. *Sociology, 23*(2), 213–234.

Women in Science (WISE). (n.d.). Retrieved January 2020, from https://www.wisecampaign.org.uk/resources/tag/statistics.

The Governance of Biomedical Science (1): Trust and the Public Understanding of Science

9

Abstract

This chapter is the first of two chapters that explore questions surrounding the building of a coherent, effective, and robust governance framework for the conduct of biomedical science research and innovation in the UK. It considers this research in terms of the governance guiding principles of social responsibility, accountability, and transparency. The chapter moves onto an assessment of the public understanding of the risks associated with innovations in bioscience and questions of public trust in the science itself. It then examines the social response to epidemics and bio-disasters and the role of government in maintaining public confidence in biomedical science innovation.

A Cautionary Tale

The bioscientist Steven Rose has illustrated an account of the struggle for scientific freedom in the former Soviet Union by describing the case of the eminent biologist, Zhores Medvedev (Rose 2019). In the late 1960s, Medvedev had sought to bring to the critical attention of the Russian public the case of the Soviet agronomist Trofim Lysenko, whose work in the 1920s had rejected Mendelian genetics in favour of an environmental explanation for the inheritance of acquired characteristics. Lysenko's non-genetic evolutionary biology was officially endorsed by the Soviet state headed by Joseph Stalin and so was subsequently integrated into an agricultural programme which attempted to socially engineer rapid improvements in plant and animal yields without accepting any role for chromosomes in seeking to environmentally engineer these new strains. This agricultural programme was a disastrous failure, leading to hundreds of thousands of deaths through famine, yet Lysenkoism, as it became known, remained the official position on genetics for many decades in the Soviet Union. This position remained despite the fact that at the time of Lysenko's original

I. Crinson, *The Biomedical Sciences in Society*,
https://doi.org/10.1007/978-981-15-9523-3_9

publication it was widely known (in the West) that his findings were based on fraudulent research. In highlighting Lysenko's errors, Medvedev was interested in much more than achieving historical revisionism, he wanted to demonstrate how a powerful and undemocratic state is able to suppress scientific facts if these did not fit with its ideological purposes. This is a view of the role of the state that is not confined to the former Soviet Union.

Medvedev's punishment for giving renewed publicity to events that had occurred nearly forty years earlier was to be confined to a psychiatric hospital. He was subsequently diagnosed as a schizophrenic on the grounds that his scientific work was concerned 'with two things at the same time, biology and society' (Rose 2019: 27). It can of course be argued that the Soviet Union was an authoritarian state and not at all comparable to the UK in the present day. That a restriction of the freedom to present critical accounts of science's role in society could never occur in a democratic and open society. Yet no coercive mechanism is required if scientists themselves do not acknowledge that they themselves have a critical role to play in the governance of science. To look beyond the confines of the laboratory and be prepared to take responsibility for both the negative and the positive impact that their research may have within a society.

The question of the accountability of science within society remains as pertinent today as it ever was. For too long, UK governments (of both political persuasions) did not seriously engage with public concerns about the social and environmental consequences of an unrestrained expansion in biomedical and biotechnological innovation. What many bioscientists may have regarded as being forward-thinking and progressive developments, many others regarded as unacceptable risks and threats to closely held communal values and ways of life. Today, a more formalised system of governance exists to ensure that the research and development practices of science are consistent with the democratic principles of social responsibility, public accountability, and effectiveness. This chapter discusses the construction of this system of governance and the challenges it now faces in a post-genomic era.

Frameworks of Science Governance

In 2009, the European Commission published a report written by its expert advisory group entitled the 'Global Governance of Science'. As the title implies, the focus was primarily with the governance of science at the global and national levels. But the interesting feature of this report is the analytical distinction it drew between what is termed 'internal' and 'external' science governance. 'Internal' governance was defined as the ways in which scientists themselves regulate the production of knowledge, through the application of systematic methodological research processes, and the processes of publishing and disseminating scientific findings. Many of these aspects were explored in Chap. 3, in the context of discussion of laboratory work and the role of epistemic scientific communities. 'External' governance was defined in the report in terms of the following five 'domains' (European Commission 2009: 11):

1. The 'upstream' funding of science and innovation usually channelled towards meeting the objectives determined by government itself.
2. The education and the encouragement of public debate surrounding the processes and products of science.
3. Establishing rules and enforcing standards of practice, for scientists and the institutions of science.
4. The formal attribution to scientific knowledge through legal means of intellectual property rights, while also ensuring open access to science knowledge.
5. The 'downstream' regulation of practice, manifested in legislation and prescriptive ethical guidelines, to check the risks and potential misuses of new developments in science and technology.

The discussion in this chapter will focus on the first two of these identified domains of external governance, which are assessed in terms of the winning of public trust and consent for the biomedical science research innovation in the UK. The final three domains are examined in Chap. 10 and relate to the construction of an enforceable system of rules and regulation over the activities of biomedical science. In relation to these last three domains, the European Commission report acknowledges that 'the most obvious and contentious form of governance involves regulation, the class of activities concerned with preventing, allowing, steering and confirming a flow of events' (European Commission 2009: 9).

In the formalised terminology of political science, the term 'governance' is usually used to denote the relationship of rule existing between a government and its citizens. The term itself only began to be widely utilised from the late 1980s onwards, complimentary to a range of social structural and cultural changes perceived at the time to be occurring within Western societies; these processes were collectively labelled 'post-modernity'. This post-modern world was depicted as one in which traditional social hierarchies were being rapidly eroded, and the command-control role of the national state increasingly displaced by new communication 'networks' facilitated by the development of innovative information technologies (but prior to the establishment of the internet). When the World Wide Web did began to develop there were many social commentators who envisaged the new social media replacing traditional top-down 'government' with new forms of digitalised governance. This vision was given expression in Prime Minister David Cameron's notion of the 'Big Society', which he first set out (albeit without much detail) on coming to power in 2010. This particular vision of governance was very much a laissez-faire one, with regulatory roles and responsibilities being gradually replaced by emergent self-organised civic networks. But this was a vision that never came close to being fulfilled. In large part because the post-modernist notion of a networked democracy ('e-democracy') was a self-constructed myth which overplayed the extent to which traditional hierarchies of power and authority had been undermined (Davies 2011: 2). Governments have continued to govern and wield substantial amounts of executive power. But it is quite possible to think about changing relationships of political and social power in terms of a continuum rather than as an absolute. It is on this basis that a much more context-bound analysis (as opposed to the social constructions of post-modernism) of the emergence of new forms of governance over the activities of science can best be understood.

Historically an informal set of arrangements existed between the government and the institutions of science that has been termed the 'social contract'. This 'contract' required the government to provide the necessary funding for science research to go ahead largely without strings attached, while the major institutions of research agreed to advance technical and scientific progress in accordance with the needs of the country. In practice, this informal separation of responsibilities was never quite as complete as some nostalgic critics now claim (Brown 2009: 17). The catalyst that led on to the ending of this informal arrangement occurred in 1996 and subsequently became known as the 'BSE crises'. This followed the establishment of a clear link between Bovine Spongiform Encephalopathy (BSE), a disease that was then affecting cattle on a large scale, and what had been up to that point, an unexplained rise in the incidence of a version of Creutzfeldt-Jacob disease (CJD), a relatively rare prion disease occurring in human brains. The linking of what had been regarded by veterinary scientists as strictly a bovine disease to human beings raised the whole question of whether variant CJD (vCJD) was a new zoonotic disease (see Glossary).

This unanticipated event shook-up the cosy relationship existing between the Department of Agriculture, Agribusiness, and the key institutions of biomedical and veterinary scientific research in this country. The government's initial response was to act defensively and engage in a public relations exercise intended to reassure the population about the safety of UK beef. However, the accumulation of pathological evidence identified prion transmission, due to the consumption of beef from cows with BSE, as the probable cause of deaths of 173 people from vCJD. This led on to the demand for, and subsequent establishment of, a public inquiry charged with examining the government's handling of the crises. The inquiry was chaired by Lord Philips, and its final report concluded that 'The government was preoccupied with preventing an alarmist over-reaction to BSE because it believed that the risk was remote. It is now clear that this campaign of reassurance was a mistake…. (t)he importance of precautionary measures should not be played down on the grounds that the risk is unproven' (Philips 2000: 266).

The 'precautionary principle' as it then became known was to assume a key role in the governance of the biomedical sciences in the UK. The principle was interpreted in a much broader way than just the narrow sense of taking 'precautions'. For it had the potential, 'to trigger and to facilitate (public) debates that went well beyond the issue of risk and into the area of responsible and socially relevant innovation' (Gee 2013: 660). The precautionary principle followed what became known the 'Democratic Model' of scientific governance, promoted by two social scientists, Alan Irwin and Peter Healey, in their submission to the House of Lords Science and Technology Select Committee in February 2000. This Committee was taking evidence in its examination of public trust in science in the wake of the BSE Crises, but prior to the publication of Lord Philips official Inquiry Report in October of the same year. Irwin and Healy argued that only a public participatory model of science could objectively evaluate the future basis of a socially, economically, and environmentally sustainable science. They argued that scientific innovation must always be predicated on a participatory process, not one in which the public are asked to merely give consent. The House of Lords Select Committee Inquiry concurred with this view and concluded that 'In modern democratic conditions, science like any other player in the public arena ignores public attitudes and values at its peril. Our call for increased and integrated dialogue with the public is intended to *secure* science's "license to practice", not to *restrict* it' (House of Lords 2000: Report Summary—Para 19—*emphasis in original*). It recommended that in future, the practices of research science should be formally scrutinised and its contribution be assessed not solely by the parameters of knowledge generation and potential economic benefits.

The New Labour government that had come to power in 1997, the year following the BSE crisis, were fully committed to 'a shift in emphasis within the governance of science, if not the imposition of an entirely novel system of control' (Gillott 2014: 52). Over the course of its first term in office, a number of major science controversies emerged that emphasised even more the requirement for a new framework of bioscience governance. These controversies included revelations about the storing and use of human tissue in biomedical research taken without consent (discussed in detail in Chap. 10), and in relation to the environment and food safety, one of the more significant developments was the test planting and potential manufacture and marketing of genetically modified (GM) foods. There were also health risk scares associated with the rapidly expanding use of mobile phones at this time, and increasingly vocalised ethical concerns about the application of new gene-editing technologies in humans. These issues 'all played a role in shaping the official approach to the governance of science as it became codified in a number of governmental and non-governmental documents' (Gillott 2014: 63).

Gray's (2004) model of governance provides a theoretical framework that sets out the 'modes' or types of levers that can be operated to bring about public accountability in the conduct of scientific research. This explanatory model was originally developed in the context of the changing relationship of medical professional governance in the UK that was also occurring at this time (late 1990s). Grey termed these modes of governance 'Command', 'Contract', and 'Communion'. The modes or forms in which governance can be structured do not constitute a hierarchy as such, but rather a range of interventions available to government. The model set out in Table 9.1 is adapted from the Grey's model and sets out the governance arrangements for biomedical science. The model provides a scaffold for thinking about the ways in which the three component aspects of governance are applied in relation to the activities of the key social actors involved in biomedical science. It should be noted that each of the three modes are not mutually exclusive, and that in practice they can work alongside each other in order to ensure the accountability of biomedical science research and innovation to the general public and to society in general.

Table 9.1 Three modes of governance (Gray 2004). Applied to biomedical science policy in the UK (as adapted by IC)

(a) **'The Command Mode'** This is governance as enacted through a set of legal and regulatory requirements that constitute a direct interventionist role for government. Typically this is achieved through primary legislation, for example, the Human Tissue Act (described in Chap. 10), combined with the establishment of formalised systems of monitoring, for example, the Human Tissue Authority or research ethics committees. The strength of this mode lies in the efficiency and effectiveness of top-down control. Its weakness lies in its lack of flexibility in the face of changing political and social circumstances.
(b) **'The Communion Mode'** This is a relationship of governance based on an appeal to a common framework of shared values and protocols. Some commentators have described this as form of 'soft' governance, as there is no 'due legal process' as in the 'Command mode'. Rather governance is constituted through an agreed set of guiding principles. One example would be the collaborative relationship that exists between the Department of Health and the pharmaceutical and biotechnology industries in the UK. This is constructed on the basis of a set of shared values concerning the necessity for companies to be more transparent about the objectives and conduct of their research and development (R&D) processes. The strength of this mode lies in this element of trust, but its weakness lies in its lack of a means for public control and accountability when, for example, these industries fail to adjust their commercial practices to meet public expectations, health needs, and normative codes of research behaviour.
(c) **'The Contract Mode'** This mode is focused on gaining consent by means of contractual inducements. For example, the government using its financial strength to award research grants or provide contracts to private or public biomedical research organisations for the development of new technological innovations on the basis of a contractual commitment (not a loose set of norms) to introduce more pro-active public engagement practices. The strength of this mode lies in the motivations to take advantage of the incentives (usually financial). The weakness of this mode is that it relies on contractual arrangements that are relatively easy to 'game' without bringing about a cultural change in the research practices of organisations. This mode also lacks the flexibility to adapt to new and changing circumstances, as any incentive to change won't necessarily occur without renegotiating changes to the specification of the original contract.

The Role of Government in Biomedical Research and Development

The establishment of a strategy for the oversight and conduct of biomedical science research does not begin and end with the construction of new constraints and regulations. Governmental systems of funding play an important role in not only achieving the objectives of current science policy, but also ensuring that frameworks of governance and accountability are adhered to. Today, research funding is not the 'no strings attached' giveaway it was in the past. It is very much linked to meeting the objectives of governmental strategy for future-orientated innovation and is particularly focused on interdisciplinary translational research. These goals are determined by the social, economic, and political priorities pertaining at the time and are frequently entangled with the infrastructural needs of industry. For example, even large-scale multi-national pharmaceutical corporations require a steady stream of biomedical science graduates to emerge from predominantly publically funded universities to become the next generation of biomedical scientists. These corporations are also increasingly looking to commercialise their knowledge-base linked to their access, facilitated by government, to the personal data sets archived by state-funded biobanks to which government provides access (discussed in detail in Chap. 10).

Historically, it was the 'Research Councils' in the UK, each responsible for one of seven main disciplinary fields of research that were the primary vehicles through which government research funding was directed. In 2018, a new quasi-autonomous body, UK Research and Innovation (UKRI), was established through primary legislation, bringing together the original research councils under one umbrella. It is the UKRI that now effectively manages the government's science budget, as well as providing regulatory advice and assurance. Expenditure for the year ending 31 March 2019 was £7.5bn (UKRI 2019), of which the bulk, £5.5 billion, was funnelled through the Department for Business, Energy and Industrial Strategy (DBEIS 2018). The UKRI umbrella also includes two new bodies, Research England and Innovate UK. Research England is responsible for providing funding to English higher education institutions for research and knowledge exchange. The funding level is determined in part by the performance of research-active academics and institutions, assessed by the parameters that are set out in the Research Excellence Framework (REF) exercise. In 2019–2020, Research England allocated £1.7 billion in research funding (Research England 2020). While Innovate UK acts as the advisory body to the government on knowledge transfer for science and technological innovation.

The government is also the largest single financial contributor to the university sector. Funding was directed through the Higher Education Funding Council for England (HEFCE) up until 2018, when it was replaced by a new body, the Office for Students (OfS). The OfS is formally an 'arms-length' regulatory body but is ultimately responsible to the Department of Education. Since 2019, the OfS has been distributing (government) funding to over 300 higher education providers under powers that formerly applied to the HEFCE. Additionally, as a member of the EU, the UK has been able to benefit from the 'Horizon 2020' research programme. Over the course of this programme, UK universities received £1.52bn of research grants, more than any other EU member state. 'Horizon Europe' succeeds 'Horizon 2020' at the end of 2020, and this programme of research is worth Euro 100 billion. However, following the Brexit referendum result, the number of UK applications fell drastically because of the future uncertainty of the UK's continued future involvement. While there were 19,127 UK applications in 2015 for Horizon 2020 research funds, this fell to 11,746 applications for Horizon Europe funding. The UK's withdrawal from the EU has raised serious concerns within the science research community about where alternative sources of funding will come from. In all likelihood the UK government will have to step-in to fill the gaps in research funding that are no longer available from the EU, there is little other option if it wants to maintain the UK's current position at the forefront of biomedical and life sciences research and innovation in the global economy.

However, there are those who have been critical of what is seen to be the disproportional percentage of UK government research and development funding directed to biomedical research over the past two decades. This has been described in a recent report as constituting a 'biomedical bubble' that threatens to unbalance the UK's research and innovation system by reducing the funding opportunities for other scientific research priorities:

> *This is not a speculative bubble...as there is far too much substance in the biomedical sciences for this. But it is a social, political and epistemic bubble, in which supporters of biomedical science create reinforcing networks, feedback loops and commitments beyond anything that can be rationalised through cost-benefit analysis. The biomedical bubble represents a risky bet on the continued success of the pharmaceutical industry, despite mounting evidence that this sector faces a deepening crisis of R&D productivity, and is cutting its own investment. And it favours a particular approach to the commercialisation of science, based on protectable intellectual property and venture capital based spinouts—despite the evidence that this model rarely works... Too often, the biomedical bubble distracts attention and draws resources away from alternative ways of improving health outcomes. Only 5 per cent of health research funding is spent on researching ways of preventing poor health.* (Jones and Wilsdon 2018: 6)

This report is written by two professors of science and reflects the concerns held by many within the natural science research field that UKRI, as the institutional body charged with the responsibility for the implementation of UK science research policy, has to move away from previous funding models. Since the first announcement of the successful completion of the sequencing of the human genome in 2003, what has been described as a 'doubling down' on biomedical research funding is seen to have occurred. That is, an ever-greater share of public funding for science being directed into an area which initially 'yielded bumper returns on investment, both financially and in terms of health gains', but there was now 'growing signs of a mismatch between disease burden and research efforts' (Jones and Wilsdon 2018: 8).

This report goes on to cite from the analysis of the UK's health research landscape produced by the UK Clinical Research Collaboration (UKCRC 2015); as of June 2020 this remains the UKCRC's most up-to-date health research analysis. The UKCRC is an independent body that brings together the NHS, research funders, industry, regulatory bodies, the Royal Colleges, patient groups, and academia in order to promote high-quality clinical research and to conduct bottom-up analysis of the impact of research grants in the health field. In 2015, 5.4% of total health research funding went to 'prevention', which included behavioural and environmental factors. 'Health services' accounted for 6.1% of funding; this covers organisational and system-wide research studies of healthcare. 'Disease management' accounted for 4% of research funding and is concerned with the experience of patients and practitioners, including self-management and palliative care. Detection and diagnosis of disease received 10.2% of research funding and focuses on the development of new biomarkers and new diagnostic methods. But the bulk of funding for health research, some 52%, was allocated to basic biomedical science, with a further 22.7% devoted to translational biomedical science. Funders have different emphases, but in total around 81% of the total spending of the research councils and medical research charities fell into areas dominated by basic and translational biomedical research in 2015 (UKCRC 2015—cited in Jones and Wilsdon 2018: 17).

In this context, Jones and Wilsdon pose the question of what is the mechanism that determines how the supply of research funding is matched to the demand for its results? They argue that this can no longer be a question of research priorities being effectively set by an elite group of bioscientists and other interested parties. Increasingly, the expectations of the public, who through direct taxation essentially fund this research, are that biomedical research should be directly addressing the health needs of the population as a whole rather than more esoteric concerns. To focus on research questions that are academically interesting to biomedical scientists but not directly relevant to clinicians and patients can they argue, be characterised as a form of 'research waste' (2018: 19). Jones and Wilsdon conclude their report with a rejoinder to the newly (in 2018) established UKRI. If it is to take seriously its commitments 'to equality, diversity and inclusion the UKRI will need to reflect on the contours of the biomedical bubble, its effects on resource allocations, and on the models and assumptions that shape priorities' (2018: 49). This last point references the need to ensure a more plural system of governance that involves an inclusive range of inputs to the research funding decision-making processes. This takes us on to a discussion of how and why the landscape of public engagement with biomedical scientific research changed so radically in a relatively short period of time.

The Public Engagement with Science

Historically, scientists have rushed to share their science with the public at times when they feel that their own enterprise is under threat. Claims that the public are uniquely the intended beneficiaries of public-understanding-of-science activities have often been disingenuous. (Gregory 2001)

The 'Public Understanding of Science' (PUS) is a self-entitled research field that has existed for some three decades or more. Its development should be understood in the context of much longer history of attempts to grapple with the question of establishing a balance between the methods of empirical science and public 'common sense' that is found within the philosophy of science. That is the question of whether there can be any continuity between the ways in which scientists and lay members of the public think about and understand the natural world that surrounds them? Or whether there is an unbridgeable epistemic chasm between both groups. As the editor of the academic journal, *Public Understanding off Science*, has noted: '(C)ommon sense is many things to many people. However, for public understanding of science research, *common sense is the contested territory*' (Bauer 2009a: 378—italics in original).

The publication in 1985 of a report produced by the Royal Society, the UK's oldest scientific institution (it immodestly describes itself as 'as the foremost learned scientific society in the country') entitled '*The Public Understanding of Science*' (more commonly referred to as the Bodmer Report) is widely held to represent the birth of the PUS movement in Britain. This report was produced at a time when science funding was being squeezed (for neither the first nor the last time), and as a result many scientists were leaving the UK to work in US research institutions and universities (euphemistically known as the 'brain drain' at the time). The Royal Society brought together a committee of unelected but distinguished scientists, 'who believed that the root of the problem was that society as a whole simply did not value science' (Gregory 2001). This committee's task was 'to review the nature and extent of public understanding of science in the United Kingdom and its adequacy for an advanced democracy; to review the mechanisms for effecting public understanding of science and technology and its role in society; [and] to consider the constraints upon the processes of communication and how they might be overcome' (The Bodmer Report 1985: 6). The report's diagnosis was that a 'public deficit' in science knowledge existed in the UK, which had to be bridged in order to retain public trust in science.

In accounting for this 'public deficit' in science knowledge, the Bodmer Report pointed to failures within the education system, but also commented on the role of the mass media in perpetuating ignorance and myths. The recommendations of the report in relation to the formal education system were that all children up to the age of 16 should follow a broad-based science curriculum which should include grounding in statistical knowledge. At that time, pupils could still opt-out from undertaking science in favour of vocational subjects such as metal and woodworking. The report also urged that the post-16 curriculum be widened so that 'no pupil at school should be allowed to take only Arts, or only science subjects'. Many of these recommended changes were subsequently incorporated into a new national curriculum for 5 to 16 year olds, enacted through the Education Reform Act of 1988, and which remains to this day. The Report also recognised the existence of science knowledge deficit not just among the general public, but also among politicians and industrialists who were urged to seek the advice of scientists on scientific and technological issues. This was seen to be necessary if the UK economy was to remain competitive. In relation to the mass media, the diagnosis of the Report was as follows:

> *The scientific community traditionally regards the mass media with some suspicion and is, on the whole, ignorant of the way they work and the nature of their constraints. The more 'popular' sections of the media, on the other hand, too often make relatively little effort to discuss science in anything other than a superficial and mostly sensational way, and do not generally understand the nature of the scientific enterprise. These attitudes need to be changed.* (Bodmer Report 1985: 21)

It was on this basis that the Report emphasised the need for scientists themselves to learn how to be more effective in communicating their research 'and consider it their duty to do so' (Bodmer Report 1985: 32). The publication of the Bodmer Report led to the establishment of the 'Committee on the Public Understanding of Science', which involved the participation of the British Association for the Advancement of Science (BAAS), the Royal Institution, and the Royal Society. The goal for this committee was to bring about a cultural change in the attitude of scientists and encourage greater involvement in public outreach activities. Two main types of academic public engagement were recommended. The first involved debunking myths held by the public about scientific research and its application. This was based on the assumption that 'false ideas' create public complacency and therefore potential harm. The Report did though recognise that newspapers and TV (the two mains forms of mass information in the 1980s, outside of the formal education system) required that detailed scientific information be presented in a more newsworthy form, which inevitably led to a reductionism of the science. However, the News Press were seen as compounding this simplification: '(B)y the inevitable choice of sensational news items, often either catastrophes or "breakthroughs"...(T) he scientist does not want always to be represented by such items. The catastrophes do not, fortunately, represent everyday scientific activities, and the supposed "breakthroughs" are often false alarms. Science as such is rarely news' (Bodmer Report 1985: 21). The second recommendation involved targeting interventions that raised the public image and profile of science. In short, for scientists to work to intensify the public's engagement with science in general, ultimately for the greater good of society (Bauer 2009a: 380).

However, the blame for a public knowledge deficit could not all be laid at the door of the education system and the mass media, scientists themselves were not averse to deploying a reductionist discourse when they wanted to gain publicity for their research. For example, the use of the notion of the 'gene for' analogy to explain a particular behaviour or mental health problem was seen by some scientists to have an attractive simplicity for the public. The view of some scientists being that, 'a simple hereditarian Mendelian account of how an allele for a particular single-gene disorder is acquired can sometimes provide quite an acceptable explanation of disease' (Barnes and Dupré 2008: 143). But this amounted to complicity with a simplistic and deterministic account of genes as fundamental to our future life, rather in the same way as fortunes are 'read' from the stars by astrologers (neatly termed 'astrological genetics' in the PUS literature). Playing the game of genetic reductionism has in practice turned out to be a hostage to fortune for biomedical science research.

Irwin and Wynne (1996), two prominent STS academics (Alan Irwin was also directly involved in promoting the 'Democratic model' of public accountability discussed), were early critics of this deficit model of public understanding. They argued that it not only depreciated the complexity of lay knowledge of science, but was also predicated on a circular self-fulfilling prophecy. That is, if the public are seen to be a priori deficient in knowledge then they cannot be trusted to participate in science innovation decision-making processes, but that mistrust of the public by scientists will then be paid back in kind. These negative public attitudes then re-confirm the assumption of scientists that the public are not to be trusted (Bauer 2009b: 5). In opposition to this deficit model, Irwin and Wynne proposed what is variously known as the 'Science-in-Society' or 'Public Dialogue' model of public engagement, which regarded the 'common sense' views of the public as a resource, a public asset: '(T)he past investment of traditions, local knowledge, social capital and values that needs to be handled with care and respect because people's life-worlds are at stake' (Bauer 2009a: 381). The role advocated for PUS research was to chart and draw the public attention to the many unpredictable and controversial events that arise due to unrestrained scientific and technological developments. In these controversies, 'the common sense of community manifests itself... as a situated recalcitrance and resistance towards an exclusive and impatient scientific expertise' (Bauer 2009a: 381). The position held by many scientists at the time was to dismiss public concerns about research innovation as simply reflecting a set of conservative and short-sighted vested interests or even irrational anxiety. Yet, this was seen by many PUS academics to be a mistaken strategy: '(M)any scientific and technological developments are intrinsically uncertain, saturated by exuberance and imagination when the real impacts still need to be defined and monitored; and here public opinion is an asset, has a role to play and must be mobilized in controversial debates' (Bauer 2009a: 381).

In summary, the last twenty years or so have seen a shift from the deficit model of public understanding which asserted that the public needed to be educated so that they can learn to trust science and its institutions, through to the gradual recognition that the public do possess important local knowledge as well as the capacity to understand technical information sufficiently to participate in policy decisions (Bucchi and Trench 2016: 154).

Techno-Scientific Innovation and Risk

Nearly three decades ago, the German sociologist Ulrich Beck (1992) identified what he saw as an important shift occurring in the public perception of the social and environmental impact of scientific 'progress', which he termed the 'reflexivity of risk'. Beck recognised this shift as reflecting, at least in part, the increasing prominence of environmental concerns as reflected in the 'Green' activism that was beginning to gain strong public support in Germany from the late 1980s onwards, and to challenge the authority of the scientific experts, initially in relation to public concerns about the safety of nuclear power. This was the background to what Beck described as the emergence of the 'risk society', a new and distinct period of history in which the hazardous environmental costs of industrialisation and technological development were increasingly being viewed by the public as far outweighing their benefits for society as a whole. Beck recognised this as a new cultural and social situation in which people are forced, willingly or not, to think through an uncertain future over which they have little or no control. 'Risk' was therefore not a question of people acting rationally (or not) according to expert advice, but rather of engaging with the societal cost of environmental destruction, and not ignoring it as in the past.

Beck's risk society thesis initially attracted some criticism for its overly, 'catastrophic assumptions about the implications of the supposedly novel contours of hazard and uncertainty in the contemporary age' (Green 2009: 495). But overtime the analysis gained leverage even within the science world, which increasingly recognised the necessity of bringing the public onboard to jointly address the 'risks' attached to unhindered technological development. However, in the UK, a rather different approach to establishing a public dialogue was adopted by industry with the support of government. This was a rehashed form of the 'knowledge deficit' model, a top-down approach designed to 'educate' the public about the difference between the (acknowledged) 'real' risks attached to technological innovation and what constituted an 'acceptable' scientific risk. One example of this approach was the public relations campaign mounted by Sellefield Ltd, the nuclear power generator in the UK. This was at a time when concerns were increasingly being expressed about the safety of the Thorp nuclear fuel reprocessing plant (one of several large nuclear facilities on one massive site in Cumbria in North-West England), following the discovery of a huge leak of radioactive material in 2004. An official report had found that a design error had caused the leak, but that it had also continued undetected for some time because of a complacent safety culture at the facility. This exposure was in the context of the long-term effects of radiation fallout that followed the Chernobyl Nuclear reactor explosion some twenty years earlier (Corporate Watch 2005). The public relations campaign involved the building of a visitors centre at the nuclear plant, with members of the public invited to go on guided tours of the facility and so be reassured that the safety culture had changed and any risks associated with the reprocessing were acceptable ones within the terms of the nuclear science (Temperton 2016). But as similar public relations campaigns began to be rolled-out in other high technology industries, 'it became clear that the public was anything but a homogeneous category…risk communication had to contend with the complexities of risk perception' (Engdahl and Lidskog 2014: 705).

So just what are these complexities of risk perception? Within both the psychology and sociology literature, perceived risk is closely linked to notions of 'trust'. For Georg Simmel (1990), the late nineteenth-century German philosopher and sociologist, for a person to give their 'trust' is not some cost-benefit process of rational choice based on an objective 'weighing-up of the facts'. Trust is seen to involve both relational and affective elements of a multi-layered set of social interactions. What Simmel termed 'mutual trust' is 'both less and more than knowledge' and requires a 'leap of faith' that necessarily involves taking a risk. Niklas Luhmann (1979, 2000), a fellow German sociologist and systems thinker but writing over half a century later, followed Simmel in recognising public trust as arising not from rational calculation, but as associated with making a 'risky investment'. Luhmann adopted a more systematic approach and drew an analytical distinction between 'confidence' and 'trust'. If a person has positive expectations of the behaviour of others (e.g., of scientific experts) in normal or everyday circumstances, then they can be said to be in a situation of 'confidence'. That is, they are confident that their expectations will not be disappointed in some way. The question of trust arises under different and uncertain circumstances, where there is a choice between acting and not acting on some information. An example might be the introduction of a new genetic biotechnology that is said to produce safe food products at a cheaper cost than through traditional agricultural methods. Here acting on information would be to trust what the experts tell us about the safety and benefits of the biotechnology and purchasing and consuming that product, while not trusting that information produces the opposite effect. But the relation between confidence and trust is not a simple zero-sum game in which the more public confidence there is in the benefits of, for example, a new biotechnology, then the less trust in what experts tell us is required (and vice versa); this would be to neglect the structural complexity of social systems.

Martin Bauer's view is that the more knowledgeable the public is, the less they are inclined to adopt an uncritical position and trust in the methods of science ('scientism') and the expertise of scientists; this he terms a 'utilitarian' assessment (2009b: 231). Utilitarianism is the ethical theory concerned with the basis of human action and derives from the work of the moral philosopher (and 'spiritual founder' of University College London) Jeremy Bentham who was writing in the early nineteenth century. Utilitarian philosophy asserts that when individuals are required to choose a course of action they do so on the basis of seeking to maximise the well-being (or happiness) of the greatest number in a society. John Stuart Mill drew on Bentham's concept and expanded upon the idea of social utilitarianism as the moral basis for human action in his book '*Utilitarianism*', published in 1863. Bauer sees the modern spirit of utilitarianism at work in the contemporary world when the public started to evaluate what science can achieve for them (its effectiveness), assessing its worth for the money that the public indirectly invest in science through their taxes (its value), and the potential for any untended consequences to arise from the science (its efficiency). This is the view that public consent to techno-scientific developments can necessarily only be given on a case-by-case basis, and that it can never be given unconditionally, as a 'leap of faith' (Bauer 2009b: 226). Others writing from a similar utilitarian perspective have argued that given its imprecision, the concept of risk adds nothing to this form of analysis and is indeed a barrier to 'better decision-making' that should rather be built on a rational assessment of effectiveness, efficiency, and the value attached to the proposed outcomes of a scientific development. The technical communication of 'risk' is seen as simply conflating the complexity of factors that should be treated as conceptually separate in their contribution to science decision-making and public choice (Dowie 1999, 2000—cited in Green 2009: 494). The assumption of a consistent human rationality underpinning the utilitarian model of public decision-making is a flaw, in the same way it is for models of economic decision-making (see the section on 'Neuroeconomics' in Chap. 5). But ultimately this does not matter, rational or not, it is the question of how science decisions get to be made and the level of involvement of the public in these processes that should be the concern of any social analysis.

Some evidence for Bauer's position of rational utilitarianism comes from the findings of the Eurobarometer survey (an instrument of the European Commission) entitled the 'Public perceptions of science, research and innovation', which has been conducted every five years for the past thirty years (European Commission 2014). Over several waves of interviews, a consistent finding of the survey has been that for those citizens of richer EU countries (higher on a national GDP scale), the more they knew about science the less likely they were to subscribe to the view that science was omnipotent in providing solutions to social problems. Therefore, within these 'knowledge-intensive developed societies' as they are termed in the survey, there is no guarantee that the more scientific knowledge possessed by an individual the more likely they are to trust science innovation. A recent global survey published in 2018 by the Wellcome Trust sought to explore what the public thought and felt about science. The first wave (the intention is to produce regular updates) of this 'Wellcome Global Monitor' brought together 140 nationally representative surveys in 140 languages, in which a total of more than 140,000 people were interviewed. The survey assessed public trust in science and scientists through the use of six questions.[1] The conclusions of the survey were that across the world, 18% of people have a high level of trust in scientists, 54% had a medium level of trust, and 14% have low trust. The remaining 13% of people were seen as having no opinion about how much they trust scientists in their respective countries. This global outcome is broken down into regions, so that one-third of participants from Australia and New Zealand, Northern Europe, and Central Asia had 'high' trust, while just one in ten had high trust in science in Central and South America. However, it was acknowledged that 'the statistical analysis was able to explain only 15% of the variation in people's trust in scientists, even when controlling for a number of factors, including personal background (gender, income, etc.) and other key variables' (Wellcome Trust 2018).

As is maybe apparent from the findings of the Welcome Global Monitor and the Eurobarometer survey cited above, the attempt to utilise the notion of 'trust' as the conceptual basis for understanding issues of public consent for science innovation appears to be as conceptually problematic as that of 'risk' when applied to real-world scenarios. A complex web of public understanding points to the validity of adopting a model of public consent to techno-scientific innovation built upon a more pragmatic form of analysis. Public assessments are necessarily localised and context-specific and predicated upon previous collective experiences of the degree to which the promissory visions of science played out.

Alternative Scenarios: Epidemics and Moral Panics

There is an alternative set of scenarios that can unfold when assessing public trust in science and 'expert' knowledge. This is when the normative cultural values and ways of life of a given society are threatened by unanticipated and novel events. The concept that is frequently invoked by sociologist's in such situations is that of the 'moral panic'.

Nearly half a century ago, the sociologist Stanley Cohen (1972) set out a conceptual framework continues to retain considerable traction in contemporary social analyses. The essence of the moral panic is the public reaction to media-driven narratives and representation of 'social threats'. As representations these threats can be both perceived and real, often at the same time. Threats can be new events not previously faced by a society, or they can be a 'camouflaged version of older well-known evils' (1972: 15). In considering whether a particular social phenomenon results in

[1] The Wellcome Global Monitor Survey (2018) posed the following question about trust in science and scientists: (a) How much do you trust scientists in this country? (b) In general, how much do you trust scientists to find out accurate information about the world? (c) How much do you trust scientists working in universities in this country to do their work with the intention of benefiting the public? (d) How much do you trust scientists working in universities in this country to be open and honest about who is paying for their work? (e) How much do you trust scientists working for companies in this country to do their work with the intention of benefiting the public?

moral panic, Cohen argues that two factors should be taken into consideration, 'disproportionality' and 'volatility' (Cohen 1999: 587). Disproportionality relates to levels of public rationality and the question of whether the congruence and appropriateness of the response of the public authorities is warranted by a particular event, threat, behaviour, or risk. The issue of volatility is concerned with whether the threat in question goes beyond what the media (not the general public) would regard as being within the normal range of what is considered to be the 'news' (Cohen 1999: 589). If it does go beyond the normal range, then the 'panic' component comes into effect. As 'drama, emergency and crisis; exaggeration; cherished values threatened; an object of concern, anxiety and hostility; evil forces or people to be identified and stopped' (Cohen 1999: 588). While the constituents of 'panic' are clear enough, whether the threat itself can be labelled a 'moral' issue may not be immediately self-evident.

The concept of pubic risk and moral panic are closely connected in social history. The more obvious examples would be fear of rising crime and violence, sexual exploitation of vulnerable people, the use of illicit drugs by young people, to which can be added threats to health arising from the various epidemics that have occurred in recent times. For Cohen, the question of morality arising out of events that occur in the political realm is quite distinct from those that arise from events in the social realm. This is why, for example, he has described the public response to the political handling of the 'BSE crises' (described above) as not being a 'classic' moral panic (1999: 589). Cohen's justification for this view is that while the BSE crisis certainly produced volatility in the media news coverage, the public response was focused on the failure of politicians to meet their responsibilities to protect the public when they played down the risk of bovine to human disease transmission. The incidence of vCJD linked to BSE never reached anything like the epidemic proportions that were initially feared, so that public focus never spilled over into a full-scale panic.

However, there are plenty of examples of the media and other elements of what might be termed the 'cultural discourse', constructing a narrative of public health risk that quickly moves beyond the issue of the political handling of a crisis to become a classic moral panic. The history of HIV/AIDS in the UK has been extensively researched and written about in terms of it being such an example of a moral panic. HIV/AIDS first emerged in the early 1980s in Western Europe and North America, and the early years of the epidemic was strongly associated in the public consciousness with two social groups who had a long-standing experience of social stigmatisation and discrimination, male homosexuals, and IV drug users. The panic that ensued was a combination of pre-existing moral fear of the lifestyles represented by these social groups and the irrational fear that all were infected with a 'killer disease'. Hence the notion of the 'Gay Plague' that was current at the time. Many young people who were dying from Aids, were at the same time experienced social ostracisation and disdain, often whipped-up by a largely homophobic national press. Initially this moral panic even manifested itself in the negative response of certain sections of the health care system, both in the USA and in the UK, to those living with HIV/Aids. Eventually, the panic began to dissipate in the UK following the direct intervention (reluctantly at first) of the government, which conducted an informed and non-moralistic public health awareness campaign. This initiative emphasised the risks of transmission attached to all forms of unprotected sexual contact, so that acquiring the virus was not limited to easily identifiable 'at-risk' groups; the virus having many modes of transmission and holding no social prejudices.

The example of MMR vaccination resistance in the UK in the late 1990s (and ongoing) is another example of a perceived threat generating unreasonable public anxieties. In this case the moral panic was directed at a national vaccination programme designed to build herd-immunity from a range of childhood infections. The moral panic first developed amongst parents of young children following the publicity given to a research paper published in the medical journal, *The Lancet*, by the now discredited researcher Andrew Wakefield. This research paper purported to offer evidence supporting a link between autism and the Measles, Mumps, and Rubella (MMR) vaccine given to all children at around the age of 12 months (MMR1) and then again at age 5 (MMR2). The paper was subsequently withdrawn by the editor of the journal, but by then the cat had been let out of the bag, so to speak. Wakefield's subsequent unsupported accusation that the medical establishment were conspiratorially withholding vital information from parents was expanded upon in certain national newspapers associated with an 'anti-expert' and anti-elitist political agenda. This could be seen to be an example of the 'risk society' hitting back, but unfortunately the public response was based on a completely false set of scientific correlations.

The major institutions of biomedical science and the medical profession, under the guidance of the government, subsequently attempted to reverse, what by the beginning of the new millennium had become a popularist anti-vaccination movement ('anti-vaxers') in the UK that went beyond the Wakefield MMR-autism link to include all forms of vaccination. The impact of this movement, although representing only a small minority of parents (but a much larger proportion in the USA), was nevertheless sufficiently large enough in numbers to seriously erode the public health goal of building herd-immunity for many common childhood illnesses. The 2019 statistics for UK childhood vaccination show that for diphtheria, tetanus, pertussis, polio, and Haemophilus Influenza type b (in shorthand—DTaP/IPV/Hib), there had been a decline in vaccination coverage for all ages. This was also the case for MMR1 coverage which had dropped below the 95% target rate, as was also the case for MMR2 (NHS 2019). In the Spring of 2019, the head of NHS England, Simon Stevens, warned that views of "vaccination deniers" were continuing to gain traction and constituted a "fake news" movement (BBC News—*Vaccination deniers gaining traction, NHS boss warns*—1st March 2019). The moral panic around childhood vaccinations lingers on, now not so much perpetuated by mainstream newspapers but through a now globalised digital social media that is almost impossible to control by traditional instruments of state governance.

A third example of a moral panic linked to a medical 'crises' is the rising levels of adult and child obesity. Epidemiologists and other biomedical scientists now routinely represent the exponential increase in the prevalence of obesity in Western societies as an 'epidemic', a biological 'fact' that is endangering the collective health of the population. Yet the focus of STS research is less on the social reasons for these increasing levels of obesity and more on the response of the experts and government to what is conceived of as moral panic. What is identified as a top-down imposition of a collective stigma on all those identified as 'obese' is seen to arise from the uncritical application of the 'Body Mass Index' (BMI), an archetypal biomedical technical construct. So that it is argued that 'obesity is being constructed by moral entrepreneurs as a way of taking or maintaining power by scapegoating those labelled obese' (Patterson and Johnson 2012: 280). The 'moral entrepreneurs' being the public health experts and institutions of government, who have framed obesity as a pathological condition arising primarily from failures of individual health behaviour requiring professional intervention. The social and economic factors that play such an important role in the increasing proportion of people across the globe labelled as obese are frequently downplayed in this narrative, in favour of one that apportions the blame onto individuals and identified 'at-risk' social groups. While the 'medicalisation' (see Glossary) of 'problematic' body weight may not be overly driven by a desire to stigmatise individuals it has that precise effect. The media did not construct an obesity epidemic out of thin air, it drew on the constructions of biomedical science; 'filtering the understanding of these prompts through their own analytic lens…sensationalising obesity as a disease to be feared, and a contagion to avoid' (Patterson and Johnson 2012: 282).

There are some important analytic differences between what can be termed 'conventional' moral panics and the moral panics that are associated with the social experience of viral epidemics. Conventional moral panics are those associated with the fear of crime or some large-scale breaching of normative codes of behaviour, as discussed above. They are usually localised epiphenomena with an impact that is more symbolic than actual. But viral moral panics 'typically involve efforts to use morality to regulate public behaviours' (Ungar 2016: 349), as indicated in the discussion of obesity above. However, as unpredictable events unfold in the context of a public health epidemic, government and health experts as the 'guardians of public safety' can sometimes overreact and lose control over the moral panic they have wittingly or unwittingly unleashed. And, from this situation of irrationality can 'converge' a range of other long-standing disagreements and opposition to top-down authority. This state of affairs can easily lead onto resistance to the recommended courses of action and behaviour designed to safeguard public health—witness the resistance of many in the USA to wearing facemasks during the Covid-19 crises. Gilman (2010) makes this point in her discussion of the moral panic that accompanied the WHO announcement of a global H1N1 influenza ('Avian flu') pandemic in 2009. While the terms 'epidemic' and 'pandemic' are strictly speaking the technical terms of epidemiological science, 'they also have a strong metaphorical use in terms of the unfettered spread of deadly and uncontrolled diseases and have always had social and emotional consequences' (Gilman 2010: 1866). The H1N1 influenza pandemic may not have turned out to be the global threat to life that it was initially thought to represent, yet 'the power of the threat and the attendant panic was real' (Gilman 2010: 1867).

Public health pronouncements have to be carefully constructed in an epidemic, for it is easier to generate a moral panic than it is to disseminate useful information about the transmission of a virus. Equally, the failure of the authorities to act effectively and efficiently, 'whether due to disregard or incompetence, readily shades into a sense of moral and criminal negligence, especially when the consequences are grave' (Ungar 2016: 355). The 2020 Covid-19 pandemic has produced many of the viral moral panic outcomes that are described above, but on a much larger scale than anything previously experienced, certainly since the influenza pandemic of 1918. Unlike other types of natural disasters and community traumas, viral pandemics require the isolation of a large proportion of the population. The impact on the psychosocial experiences of individuals who have experienced physical isolation from local and work communities during the pandemic are yet to be fully understood. Sun et al.'s (2020) study of the impact of Covid-19 pandemic on those living in China where the virus first appeared, draws on interviews with college students and identified the following themes:

> *Participants described excessive internet and smartphone usage as a common avoidance coping for anxiety, disrupted social life, and insomnia. Participants also noted that smartphone/internet-based avoidant coping "feeds off" anxiety and insomnia-related issues (e.g., excessive news watching on COVID-19 could further fuel one's anxiety). In addition, due to the lack of early transparency by authorities, people may experience anxiety and distrust toward their medical system. As such, they may be particularly vulnerable to misinformation and un-founded conspiracy theories about COVID-19.* (Sun et al. 2020: S26)

In the UK, there is also evidence that misinformation, often fuelled by exaggerated headlines in the news and social media have reinforced pre-existing health-related fears and phobias. There is among several other seemingly irrational behaviours, an insipid xenophobia directed towards Chinese people, which draws on long-established tropes concerning the 'yellow peril' that go back to the nineteenth century. The concept of the moral panic and the role played by the authorities and the media in invoking fear within a population while seeking to control an epidemic, whether considered or not, points to how alternative scenarios concerning the building of public trust in science expertise and innovation can all too easily play out in practice.

Chapter Summary: Key Points

- *The governance of science is concerned with ensuring social justice, public accountability, and effectiveness.*
- *There exists a balance or mosaic of modalities of governance, rather than the one overarching set of regulatory mechanisms in relation to biomedical science research.*
- *The UK government utilises a variety of funding vehicles to assert control over the direction of science research and training.*
- *The Bodmer Report published in 1985 marked the birth of the 'Public Understanding of Science' movement, its objective being to engage with and build public trust in science.*

- *The education system, mass media, and scientists themselves are seen to have an important top-down role in countering the 'deficit' in public understanding of science.*
- *An alternative 'Public Dialogue' model of public engagement in science regards the public's 'common sense' as a resource, a public asset.*
- *The 'Risk Society' concept examines the cultural context in which people are confronted by the social and environmental costs of unregulated technological development.*
- *Science and technology industries have more recently sought to change public risk perceptions of their activities by drawing a line between 'acceptable' and 'real' risks.*
- *The constructs of 'risk' and 'trust' dominant the public response to science literature, but bring with them considerable conceptual difficulties when applied to actual events.*
- *Both governments and media have been complicit in contributing to narratives of public health risk that all too easily lead on to from to a classic moral panic.*
- *There are some important analytic differences between 'conventional' moral panics and the moral panics that are associated with the social experience of viral epidemics.*
- *The 2020 Covid-19 pandemic has resulted in many outcomes that can be associated with a classic viral moral panic, but on a much larger scale than anything previously experienced since the influenza pandemic of 1918.*

Bibliography

Barnes, B., & Dupré, J. (2008). *Genomes and What to Make of Them*. London: University of Chicago Press.

Bauer, M. (2009a). Editorial. *The Public Understanding of Science, 18*(4), 378–382.

Bauer, M. (2009b). The Evolution of Public Understanding of Science—Discourse and Comparative Evidence. *Science, Technology and Society, 14*(2), 221–240.

Beck, U. (1992). *Risk Society: Towards a New Modernity*. London: Sage.

Bodmer Report. (1985). *The Public Understanding of Science*. London: The Royal Society. Retrieved September 2017, from https://royalsociety.org/~/media/Royal_Society_Content/policy/publications/1985/10700.pdf.

Brown, M. (2009). *Science in Democracy: Expertise, Institutions, and Representation*. Cambridge, MA: MIT Press.

Bucchi, M., & Trench, B. (2016). Science Communication and Science in Society: A Conceptual Review in Ten Keywords. *Technoscienza, 7*(2), 151–168.

Cohen, S. (1972). *Folk Devils and Moral Panics*. London MacGibbon and Kee.

Cohen, S. (1999). Moral Panics and Folk Concepts. *Paedagogica Historica, 35*(3), 585–591.

Corporate Watch. (2005). *Newsletter*, 21. Retrieved from https://corporatewatch.org/content/newsletter-21-3-its-official-no-dark-machiavellian-conspiracy-new-nuclear-power.

Davies, J. (2011). *Challenging Governance Theory*. Bristol: Policy Press.

Department of Business, Energy and Industrial Energy. (2018). *The Allocation of Funding for Research and Innovation*. London: BEIS.

Dowie, J. (1999). Communication for Better Decisions: Not About 'Risk'. *Health, Risk & Society, 1*, 41–53.

Dowie, J. (2000). A Risky Decision: Managing without Risk. *Risk Management: An International Journal, 2*, 51–73.

Engdahl, E., & Lidskog, R. (2014). Risk, Communication and Trust: Towards an Emotional Understanding of Risk. *The Public Understanding of Science, 23*(6), 703–717.

European Commission. (2009). *Global Governance of Science—Report of the Expert Group on Global Governance of Science*. EUR 23616 EN. Luxembourg: Publications Office of the European Union.

European Commission. (2014). *Special Eurobarometer 419—Public Perceptions of Science, Research and Innovation*. Brussels: European Commission.

Gee, D. (2013). *More or Less Precaution? Late Lessons from Early Warnings: Science, Precaution, Innovation*. Copenhagen: European Environment Agency.

Gillott, J. (2014). *Bioscience, Governance and Politics*. Basingstoke: Palgrave.

Gilman, S. (2010). The Art of Medicine: Moral Panic and Pandemics. *The Lancet, 375*, 1866–1867.

Gray, A. (2004). Governing Medicine: An Introduction. In A. Gray & S. Harrison (Eds.), *Governing Medicine: Theory and Practice* (pp. 5–20). Maidnhead: Open University Press.

Green, J. (2009). Is It Time for the Sociology of Health to Abandon 'Risk'? *Health, Risk and Society, 11*(6), 493–508.

Gregory, J. (2001). Public Understanding of Science: Lessons from the UK Experience. *SciDevnet*. Retrieved September 2016, from http://www.scidev.net/global/communication/feature/public-understanding-of-science-lessons-from-the.html.

House of Lords. (2000). Select Committee on Science and Technology, Third Report—*Science and Society*. Retrieved from http://www.publications.parliament.uk/pa/ld199900/ldselect/ldsctech/38/3801.htm.

Irwin, A., & Wynne, B. (1996). *Misunderstanding Science? The Public Reconstruction of Science and Technology*. Cambridge: Cambridge University Press.

Jones, R., & Wilsdon, J. (2018). *The Biomedical Bubble: Why UK Research and Innovation Needs a Greater Diversity of Priorities, Politics, Places and People*. London: NESTA.

Luhmann, N. (1979). *Trust and Power*. Chichester: Wiley.

Luhmann, N. (2000). Familiarity, Confidence, Trust: Problems and Alternatives. In G. Diego (Ed.), *Trust: Making and Breaking Cooperative Relations*. Oxford: University of Oxford.

NHS. (2019). Childhood Vaccination Coverage Statistics—England: 2019–20. https://digital.nhs.uk/data-and-information/publications/statistical/nhs-immunisationstatistics/england---2019-20.

Patterson, M., & Johnson, J. (2012). Theorizing the Obesity Epidemic: Health Crisis, Moral Panic and Emerging Hybrids. *Social Theory & Health, 10*, 265–291.

Philips, N. L. (2000). *The BSE inquiry. Volume 1, Findings and Conclusions*. London: Stationary Office.

Research England. (2020). Annual Funding Allocations 2019–20. Retrieved January 2020, from https://re.ukri.org/finance/annual-funding-allocations/annual-funding-allocations-2019-20/.

Rose, S. (2019, July 18). Pissing in the Snow. *London Review of Books, 41*(14).

Simmel, G. (1990). *The Philosophy of Money*. London: Routledge.

Sun, S., Lin, D., & Operario, D. (2020). Need for a Population Health Approach to Understand and Address Psychosocial Consequences of COVID-19. *Psychological Trauma: Theory, Research, Practice, and Policy, 12*(S1), S25–S27.

Temperton, J. (2016). Inside Sellafield: How the UK's Most Dangerous Nuclear Site Is Cleaning Up Its Act. *Wired*, 17 September 2016.

UK Clinical Research Collaboration—UKCRC. (2015). *UK Health Research Analysis 2014*. London: UKCRC.

UK Research and Innovation—UKRI. (2019). *Annual Report and Accounts 2018–19*. HC207. Swindon: UKRI.

Ungar, S. (2016). Is This One It? Viral Moral Panics. In C. Krinsky (Ed.), *The Ashgate Research Companion to Moral Panics* (pp. 349–366). London: Routledge.

Wellcome Trust. (2018). Wellcome Global Monitor 2018. Retrieved January 2020, from https://wellcome.ac.uk/reports/wellcome-global-monitor/2018.

The Governance of Biomedical Science (2): Regulation, Biodata, and Big Data

10

Abstract

This chapter is the second of the two chapters exploring the governance of biomedical science. It draws on three case studies in assessing the reasons why regulatory mechanisms were introduced to govern the conduct of biomedical science research in the postmillennial period. The discussion then moves on to an examination of the role and function of biobanks as repositories of human biological material and personal data, as they have taken on a greater prominence as resource for the genomic research. It examines developments in bioinformatics, and the influential role it now plays in the processing and analysis of genomic 'big data'.

Introduction

The post-millennial period has been characterised by what many political commentators have identified as the emergence of what has been termed a 'regulatory state' in the UK. This conception is linked with the establishment of regulatory agencies charged with oversight over the activities of privatised former state industries. For example, Ofcom for telecommunications, Ofgem for electricity and gas markets, and ONR for Nuclear power generations. These developments have been mirrored in the attempts to impose greater top-down control over the internal activities of state institutions themselves. In relation to the national health care system, this process would include the re-organisation of the General Medical Council (GMC), the ending of the self-regulation of the medical profession and the introduction of new systems of clinical accountability designed to limit the relative decision-making autonomy of doctors. In the national education system, this regulatory approach

I. Crinson, *The Biomedical Sciences in Society*,
https://doi.org/10.1007/978-981-15-9523-3_10

would be reflected in the processes through which the Department of Education has accrued greater powers to enforce national curriculum standards and assessment in schools and colleges, effectively ending their day-to-day management by locally accountable education authorities. In relation to science and specifically biomedical research, the creation of new regulatory regimes has seen an end to the informality characterised by the close bonds that once existed between the top figures in the key institutions of science and senior civil servants and politicians. Far from the national state being 'hollowed-out' in the face of a globalised economy, as was being predicted by many political analysts back in the 1990s, today national states such as that in the UK 'have continued to grow as regulators as they have contracted as providers (of services)' (Braithwaite 2013).

The concerns of this chapter are centred on the social, ethical, and political concerns that led to the building of a formalised system of governance over the course of the past two decades to regulate the conduct of biomedical science research in the UK. The chapter begins with an assessment of three case studies of regulation, each of which assesses a significant legislative milestone in the development of the system of governance. This is followed by an exploration of the role and function of biobanks as they have become a primary resource for genomic disease research. This is followed by a discussion of the social and bioethical issues that have arisen as a consequence of the commercial exploitation of personal health data. Finally, the impact of bioinformatics and the application of computational methodologies to 'mine' a network of health data sets are assessed in terms of its implications for traditional ways of 'doing' biomedical science.

Three Case Studies in the Regulation of Research

> *Fundamentally, there was a social and ethical time bomb waiting to go off. It is no surprise that the explosion of anger when it came was huge. The cause lay in two conflicting attitudes. For the parents of a recently deceased child, human material, certainly substantial specimens such as organs and parts of organs and even smaller samples, are still thought of as an integral part of the child's body and thus still the child. For the pathologist and clinician the material is regarded as a specimen or an object. it is dehumanised.* (Kennedy 2001)

The excerpt above is taken from the 2001 report of the official Inquiry led by Professor Ian Kennedy into a paediatric heart surgery 'scandal' that had occurred at the Bristol Royal Infirmary over the course of the 1990s. This public inquiry followed on from other revelations concerning the retention and use of children's organs for research without ethical permission at Alder Hay Children's Hospital in Liverpool, which in turn fuelled a growing public perception that the use of human organs in biomedical research needed to be constrained and controlled. Up until to these events, many research bioscientists had seen no ethical problem in the use of human organs, whether freshly taken from a cadaver or preserved in jars. Human organs were widely regarded in the field as purely research materials, nothing more.

Histological slides had been an integral part of medical education for over a century, and every medical school had its own pathology museum utilised as an essential teaching resource. What might have seemed a straightforward set of educational and research practices prior to the mid-1990s became much more complex and fraught after the Alder Hay and Bristol Royal Infirmary revelations.

Following the Bristol public inquiry, the Secretary of State for Health instigated a process of public consultation over a series of proposed legislative reforms, these went beyond the concerns associated with the use of retained organs (Gillott 2014: 115). The consultation process culminated in the drafting and the passing of primary legislation in 2004, from which emerged the Human Tissue Act. This legislation also established an arms-length regulatory authority, the Human Tissue Authority (HTA), legally charged with licensing research activities involved with human tissue. More broadly, the 2004 legislation combined with the regulatory agency was designed to bring about a cultural change within the institutions of biomedical and clinical science research. This required a shift from a high-handed culture of a scientific exceptionalism to the self-recognition that as institutions of science serving society, they had social and ethical responsibilities that could not be shunned when it came to using human tissue for research purposes. The Human Tissue Act had the effect of progressively replacing pre-existing professional norms of discretion and confidently, with a new set of norms based on the principle of informed consent.

The 2004 legislation established the right of individual patients and their families to determine what should happen to their biological material. This development has been described succinctly 'as a rights-based framework set against a dignitarian baseline' (Price 2009: 283—cited in Gillott 2014: 119). While others have described this regulatory process as one where 'people are no longer prepared to be the passive recipients of medical beneficence or to have themselves or their families treated merely as the "subjects" of research' (Campbell et al. 2008: 108). The case for establishing the principle of informed consent was made consistently during the passage of the Human Tissue Bill through Parliament, and as such, became known as the 'Golden Thread'. However this did stop the biomedical science community from lobbying hard in the final stages of the drafting process of the Bill to limit the impact of this Golden Thread principle. To a certain extent the community was successful in this lobbying. The final enacted legislation included a number of exceptions to the principle that informed consent was always to be a legal requirement when storing and using human tissue for research. These exceptions were: '(T)issue which is an "existing holding", i.e. it was already held before 1 September 2006; tissue which has been taken from a living person AND the researcher is not able to identify the person AND the research project is ethically approved by a Research Ethics Committee; imported human tissue' (Health Research Authority 2019—*emphasis in original*). A willingness to concede on some aspects of the principle of consent in certain circumstances reflected the desire of government to maintain its 'pro-science' position. That is, it had no intention of being seen as impeding biomedical research as long as that it continued to achieve palpable therapeutic benefits for patients:

> *Although consent has been proclaimed as the cornerstone of the UK Human Tissue legislation, the underlying rationale is essentially utilitarian. The government believes that the effect of the consent provisions will be to "help improve public confidence so that people will be more willing to agree to valuable uses of tissues and organs".* (Brownswood 2010: 26—cited Gillott 2014: 121)

Four years later in 2008, the Labour government introduced the Human Fertilisation and Embryology (HFE) Act. It had determined that human embryo and human infertility treatment research and the associated use of human gametes (reproductive cells, female ova, and male sperm) required further regulation to keep pace with the advances that had been made in human embryo research and in reproductive technologies in the intervening period since the passing of the 1990 Act of the same name. The earlier legislation was the first to establish a regulatory regime for embryo research and for infertility treatment that involved the creation of embryos outside a woman's body; all overseen by the Human Fertilisation and Embryology Authority (HFEA) that had been established at the same time. In the public consultation process that led on to the restructuring of the pre-existing legislation, the Department of Health stated that 'The (1990) Act has stood the test of time well, and is a tribute to the foresight of its creators ... The Act and the regulatory system it established have instilled public confidence in the safe and ethical use of assisted reproduction technology subject to appropriate safeguards. However, it was never expected that the Act would remain forever unchanged in this area of fast-moving science' (DoH 2005).

There were some significant differences in the consultation process that led up to the 2008 HFE legislation from that of the Human Tissue Act four years earlier. Consultation on the latter had involved the lining-up of two essentially antagonistic groups. On one side were the patient and parent groups outraged by what they saw as being the unethical use of human tissue that belonged to their loved ones. On the other side of the fence was the biomedical science community who were concerned that their research autonomy was under threat. Their primary concern was that they would now have to undertake what was perceived to be the onerous additional work of seeking consent for the use of research materials that they had always previously used without interference. In the case of the 2008 HFE legislative process, patient groups and research scientists now worked together to bring the government and the regulator (HFEA) around to view that many of the existing embryological research practices should be retained, albeit under a tougher but 'research-friendly' regulatory regime. However, outside of the patient and research groups, there were organised sections of the public that expressed strong concerns about the ethics of allowing research with hybrid/admixed embryos to go ahead (Gillott 2014: 96). The government was convinced at the time that the public could be won over to the long-term medical benefits to embryonic research, and this largely proved to be the case. These two pieces of regulatory legislation firmly established the principle of requiring informed consent for research that involved human cells and tissue.

The third case study of the regulation of biomedical science research focuses on the difficulties associated with sustaining a framework able to keep abreast with rapid developments in genome editing (see Glossary) in the field of embryo science. Three distinct types of therapeutic applications of genome editing can be identified, each of which raise different ethical concerns. These applications are (a) specific therapies involving genome-edited immune cells, for which human trials are already established; (b) 'somatic cell' editing, involving modification of adult cells in the affected tissue; and (c) 'germline' editing of sperm or egg cells that can lead on to heritable changes passed on to future generations. All three types of application are utilised within bioscience research and clinical practice, overseen by a range of regulators in the UK that include the Human Tissue Authority, the Medicines and Healthcare Products Regulatory Agency, and the Human Fertilisation and Embryology Authority.

In 2018, the UK Parliament Select Committee on Science and Technology established an investigation into the state of genomic research and genome editing governance. Their report stated the following: 'Therapies involving somatic genome editing are regulated similarly to other gene therapies, and clinical trials of such therapies have already started. The implantation of a genetically altered embryo into a woman is currently prohibited under the Human Fertilisation and Embryology Act 2008, other than under certain conditions to prevent the transmission of serious mitochondrial disease. Research involving human embryos, up to 14 days old, is permitted subject to the conditions of the Act' (Parliament UK 2018: para 102). The Select Committee investigation took evidence from various stakeholders, including the Wellcome Trust, the Association of Medical Research Charities, and Cancer Research UK. All these institutional bodies were concerned to emphasise the differences between genome editing of somatic, germ cells and embryos as well as the differences between research and clinical applications. They also all agreed that these different applications should be distinguished in any debate concerning the ethics of genome editing, as well as the need to emphasis the potential benefits of these new technologies (Parliament UK 2018: para 98). However, Professor Chris Whitty, the then Interim Government Chief Scientific Adviser, told the Select Committee that genome editing is 'an area where science cannot stray beyond what the public, as represented by Parliament, are comfortable with' (Parliament UK 2018: para 101). While the view of the Department of Health was that it did not want to undertake a review of the 14-day rule, 'there are risks in opening up that Act, because it is not about mitochondria and gene editing; it is about a lot of women's health' (Parliament UK 2018; para 104). The expressed view of the government is that they had no plans to amend the 2008 HFE Act to permit germline modifications.

But concerns have grown in recent years about research involving human genetic enhancement of various kinds being conducted in countries that lack publically accountable regulatory frameworks. Currently thirty countries, including the UK, have legislation that directly or indirectly bars germline editing. A recent comment piece in *Nature* called for a global moratorium on all clinical uses of human germline editing. The proposed moratorium would in effect be a global framework of governance, one in which nations voluntarily committed themselves to not approving the use of germline editing unless certain ethical conditions were met, in particular the transfer of an embryo to a human uterus (Lander et al. 2019: 165). The signatories to this call for a moratorium stating that 'no clinical application of germline editing should be considered unless its long term biological consequences are sufficiently understood, both for individuals and for the human species … (A) ttempting to reshape the species on the basis of our current state of knowledge would be hubris' (Lander et al. 2019: 166). Interestingly, the signatories also argued that the moratorium should be a voluntary process, on the basis that a purely regulatory agency approach would be inadequate to the task, because such agencies have 'narrow mandates' and are primarily concerned with 'safety and efficacy' (Lander et al. 2019: 167). Whatever the view of the voluntary nature of such a moratorium, the call does point to the fact that germline research is now global, and its outcomes have the potential to impact on all of humanity.

A final word in this section goes to Sheila Jasanoff. A decade prior to the call for a moratorium of genome editing she argued that greater humility needed to be shown by scientists given the ambiguity, indeterminacy, and complexity inherent in the research process: 'It is a request for research on what people value and why they value it. It is a prescription to supplement science with the analysis of those aspects of the human condition that science cannot easily illuminate. It is a call for policy analysts and policy-makers to re-engage with the moral foundations for acting in the face of inevitable scientific uncertainty' (Jasanoff 2007: 33).

The Role of Biobanks in Biomedical Research

The role played by 'biobanks' as repositories of human biological material and personal health data has come to take on a much greater prominence in biomedical research over the past decade. There has been a considerable expansion in biobanking facilities alongside the exponential growth in post-genomic research, particularly in relation to the processes of gene mapping and gene expression profiling. This process has been facilitated by new biotechnologies and the emergence of bioinformatics as a mode of data processing and analysis. Biobanks can be defined as any collection or 'biorepository' of human biological material and associated clinical data that is stored, processed, and distributed for ongoing and future scientific research. This biomaterial comprises tissue samples that include tumour tissue, cells, blood, DNA, and DNA array results; these samples are then linked with an individual's phenotypic, lifestyle, and personal social information. Biobanks rely completely upon the willingness of participants to voluntarily donate their biomaterial and personal health data, and in return, the expectation is that these institutions store and manage this material in ethically and legally legitimate ways. Biobanks can be found within or hosted by academic and research institutions, hospitals, biotechnology and pharmaceutical companies, stand-alone private companies, or charitable foundations. They may be publically or privately owned or may under joint partnership control across sector boundaries.

Biobanks can serve several distinct but often converging functions. These can include acting as a database for biomedical research; as a forensics database; as a source of information for transplantation; as a resource for therapeutics, for example, the storing of stem cells for individual or community use; and as a source of diagnostics, for example, of viral or bacterial infectious diseases. However as a rule, two main types of biobanks may be distinguished: (1) disease-orientated biobanks which collect donated material from specific groups of patients or donors and (2) population research focused which collect samples from the general population, both healthy and from those with a diagnosed disease. In practice, there is considerable overlap between these two types of facility. For example, population-based research relies upon data end-points from disease-orientated biobanks for clear delineation of phenotypes and for RNA analysis. While disease-orientated researchers need to be able to control for both population cohort effects and biological material collected at an earlier point in time, and this information can be sourced from the population-orientated biobanks (Gottweis and Petersen 2008: 6).

The typical research applications for the wide variety of biomaterial held within biobanks include the following:

- As a resource for genome-wide association studies (GWAS), seeking to identify genetic susceptibilities and their impact on individual response to pharmaceuticals, facilitating the expansion and development of precision medicine.
- As a resource for health outcome surveys in order to better understand how genetic diseases affect people as their illness progresses.
- The development of treatment options depends on carrying out research with comprehensive collections of DNA samples, collected from those affected by specific disorders.
- As a resource for a better understanding of environmental factors and population health. For example, in researching the effect of environmental factors in asthma and diabetes, or how the misuse of alcohol affects the development of diseases in different individuals, or in identifying key environmental factors in epigenetic change.
- As a community resource to better understand the local spread of childhood infectious diseases.
- In improving law enforcement through the matching of DNA samples to aid in the prosecution and conviction of criminals (this is not strictly a biobank but a 'forensic DNA database').

Biobanks can range in size, from specialised disease-orientated repositories that contain biodata from just a few thousand individuals to massive population-based biobanks containing data from as many as a million or more donors. For example, the 'UK Biobank', a registered charity primarily funded by the Medical Research Council and the Wellcome Trust, has recruited a 'prospective cohort' of some 500,000 individuals aged between 40 and 69 over the course of the period 2006–2010. The mission of the UK Biobank is to act as a resource for any health-related research conducted in the public interest, including the investigation of the genetic, environmental, and lifestyle determinants of a wide range of diseases of middle age and later life. Data on participants' lifestyles, environment, medical history, and physical measures, along with biological samples are collected, and their health monitored at regular intervals over the long term. These objectives are achieved principally through linking the biobank to electronic health records (UK Biobank 2019). UK Biobank is also subject to a set of governance arrangements that followed a process of public consultation. The consultation involved the establishment of focus group discussions as a form of public opinion sampling organised by a market research company. While this process hardly constituted a full and transparent public consultation, it did occur in the early 2000s at a relatively early period in the development of science governance frameworks in the UK. The decision was also made at this early stage to allow commercial companies engaged in profit-making research access to the voluntary donated biobank materials. There was a very mixed response to this decision during the focus group consultation process, but this decision went ahead anyway. We will now explore this question of the commercialisation of biomaterial below in greater detail.

In most EU member states, biobanks are subject to inspections by various statutory bodies, which in the UK would include the HFEA and the HTA. They are also subject to less formal accountability mechanisms, including advisory boards, forms of professional guidance, and internal governance policies. However, unlike other areas of scientific research practice, including the use of personal data, there remains no European Union-wide harmonised system of regulation governing the use of human samples and health data by biobanks. The EU regulatory framework that currently exists spans a number of areas of EU law, including general data protection regulations (GDPR), clinical trials, and tissue regulation. But in essence, it is only national laws that apply to the use of human tissue in research in the EU member states, including different licensing regimes, individual rights, biobank-specific laws, and research-specific laws. So there remains considerable scope for national legal variation (Kaye et al. 2016: 198).

Commercialising Biodata: A Challenge for Regulation

When people donate their biomaterial to biobanks, they are often contributing 'simultaneously to state and pharmaceutical interests, public and private value' (Mitchell and Waldby 2010: 336). The reality of commercialisation directly follows from the close links that exist between publically funded biobanks and private research enterprises. The involvement of private capital is often essential to the financial sustainability of public biobanks, enabling them to fully realise their research potential, which is particularly the case for small-scale, not-for-profit university or hospital-based biobanks. The motivation for commercial funders to invest in these smaller institutions is to bring together the digital data held in these facilities to create larger 'virtual' biobanks that can then become attractive platforms for profitable research (Meijer et al. 2012). Additionally, publically funded biobanks also often charge fees for access to their resources to fully leverage the commercial value of their data sets.

The potential for commercialisation raises several important ethical and legal considerations. The first concerns whether the commercial application for data use is consistent with the original informed consent given by the donors. This point will be expanded upon in the following section in terms of which bioethical principles best fit the particularities of the multiple uses made of donated material. The second issue concerns the intellectual property rights of the biobank and whether these can be safeguarded. This references the potential for commercial research companies to patent newly identified genes, thereby locking-in the knowledge generated via publically funded biobanks, into what has been termed an 'International Intellectual Property Regime' (Birch 2012: 198). The process of commercialisation can result in a fundamental contradiction for biobanks, 'between open cooperation in knowledge and privatized control and exploitation' (Birch 2012: 184). Commercialisation having the potential to undermine the moral principle of altruism that accompanies the personal donation of biomaterial which acts to serve the needs of biomedical science while at the same time contributing to the public good (Turner et al. 2013: 72). Unlike the application of biomaterial constructed in the lab such as tissue cell-lines, the use of donated tissue and personal health information depends crucially on the willingness of participant donors to be available for follow-up sampling over an extended period of time. There is therefore a case to be made that this contribution should be seen as adding an additional 'biovalue' to any commercial exploitation of biobank material (Mitchell and Waldby cited in Turner et al. 2013: 74).

The attitudes and beliefs that underlie the decisions of members of the public to voluntarily donate their biomaterial and personal health data are relatively under-researched. But one example of research in this field is a qualitative study that involved focus group discussions carried out in Norway in 2013. This study found that members of the public were comfortable with donating their personal biomaterial but only in terms of a 'gift relationship'. That is, a donation with no expectation of financial gain, but on the basis that the biobank would then be under a moral obligation to use this 'gift' to benefit all, not for commercial gain. The Norwegian study found that financial gain was not seen as wrong per se by the participants, but that it was the commercialisation of a 'gift' that was perceived to be wrong because it led to an 'unjust' financial gain. In other words, a clear distinction was made by the study participants between the concern for 'dignity' in donation and the concern for 'justice' in the use of their tissue samples (Steinsbekk et al. 2013: 158). This interesting study concludes with a summary of the participant's views: 'In a biobank setting the deed is done, a gift is given and it is the stewards' responsibilities not mine, to ensure that anonymity and professional secrecy is granted and that the promises of the project are fulfilled by utilising the resources in a proper manner' (Steinsbekk et al. 2013: 158). The concept of the 'gift relationship' actually originates from Richard Titmuss' (1970) classic work on altruistic blood donation as an example of a process that contributes to holding a society together. Titmuss' study explored why almost uniquely in the health care systems across the world at that time, the NHS operated a system of voluntary blood donation, and why this was seen to be economically, morally, and clinically superior to systems that relied on paying donors for their blood. The dangers he associated with the process of commercialisation, in the case of paying for blood donation, were seen to lead on to heightened risk of transfusion-transmitted infections.

Bioethical Principles in the Context of the Governance of Biobanks

The ethical and legal issues associated with the operation of biobanks as repositories of donated biomaterial extend to concerns about the potential for infringing privacy and personal property rights. The Human Genome Project was a notable early example of a research programme that incorporated a study of the ethical, legal, and social ('ESL') implications of the research as a core activity. These 'ESL' initiatives as they came to be known are examples of an 'internal' element of research governance designed 'to anticipate and manage societal issues, reassure publics, and maintain political legitimacy' (Hilgartner et al. 2017: 823). The ELS approach is necessarily interdisciplinary, involving the participation of social scientists and bioethicists, in addition to the biomedical scientists directing the primary programme of research. Yet despite an increase in these 'internal' governance initiatives, there inevitably remains a massive power differential between the commercial and the public organisations conducting large-scale biomedical programmes of research and the general public who are asked to participate as subjects or donors. In the past, this often meant that any ethical concerns about the conduct of a research programme were subsumed to the achievement of the overall aims.

Today in the USA, all biomedical science research is regulated through the Federal Policy for Protection of Human Research Subjects. This policy is the outcome of a process that was several decades in the making. It was the US National Commission for the Protection of Human Subjects of Biomedical and Behavioral Research that laid the groundwork for the establishment of framework for the ethical conduct of research involving human subjects. The National Commission sets out this framework in what subsequently became known as the 'Belmont Report', published in 1978. The report identified three key ethical principles (respect for persons or autonomy, beneficence, and justice) as justifying its recommendations for the adoption of an informed consent approach to research. These principles have provided the philosophical basis for the development of bioethics policies to this day. They were more fully articulated in Beauchamp and Childress' publication, 'Principles of Biomedical Ethics' published a year later (1979/2001), both authors having been members of the 1978 National Commission. This book, now in its 5th edition, has become a primary resource in any deliberation about the ethical issues underpinning the practice of clinical practice and biomedical research. The three principles set out in the original Belmont report were revised and became four:

1. Respect for autonomy: Respecting the decision-making capacities of autonomous persons. Enabling individuals to make reasoned informed choices.

2. Beneficence: The balancing of the benefits of treatment against its risks and costs. The health care professional should act in a way that benefits the patient.
3. Non maleficence: To avoid causing harm. Although all treatments have the potential to cause some harm, even if minimal, that harm should not be disproportionate to the benefits of treatment.
4. Justice: The distributing of benefits, risks, and costs fairly. This is the notion that patients in similar positions should be treated in a similar manner.

In the four decades since Beauchamp and Childress' principles were first published, questions have increasingly been asked about their over-reliance on informed consent to manifestly achieve respect for the autonomy of participants in clinical and biomedical research setting: '(I)nformed consent should not be the primary tool for preventing research subjects from harm and ensuring fairness; instead, ethics governance should ensure that subjects are not exposed to unreasonable risks or treated unjustly. To put the main burden of assessing the risks and benefits of participation on the individual subject through informed consent would indeed be unfair' (Kristinsson 2009: 612). This discussion paper goes on to cite the moral philosopher Onora O'Neill, in its assertion that reliance on just one instrument, informed consent, could resolve the issues surrounding the extent of the control that research subjects and patients should have over the amount of information they receive. The danger of being deceived or coerced is effectively limited when people 'know that they have access to extendable information and that they have given rescindable consent' (O'Neill 2003: 5—cited in Kristinsson 2009: 615).

Biobanks are in many ways unique institutions of research, and consent to participate in practice shares little in common with the clinical management of patients. The Beauchamp and Childress' principles were never designed to accommodate the very long timescales over which biomaterial can potentially be stored prior to its use in research and subsequently used for research purposes that were not anticipated at the time of donation. Biobanks also require donors to be able to retain and recall the information about the potential risks attached to the use of their biomaterial provided to them at the time of their original donation. Problems with the retention of knowledge are a well-known issue in giving consent for participation in clinical trials conducted over a much shorter duration than the timescales operated by biobanks. All these practical issues make it difficult for biobanks to fulfil the terms of informed consent. In response, Research Ethics Committees have sought to resolve at least some of these concerns by enabling biobanks to recruit participants on the basis of what is known about risk at the time the individual makes their donation (Strech 2015). This is known as the principle of 'broad consent' and authorises the use of samples and personal data for a large, vaguely defined spectrum of research aims. However, while this variant of informed consent may serve to protect the institution from any future legal challenges, it does not overcome all the concerns about the future potential for an unscrupulous use of a donor's biomaterial.

A further ethical consideration of relevance to the governance of biobanks relates to the difficulty in guaranteeing donor anonymity. The potential of biobanks lies precisely in their ability to link biomaterial to individual medical histories and other forms of personalised data and, if required, ask the individual donors to regularly update their personal information. One potential solution is to 'double code' the sample and the personal health data to the individual (Hansson 2009). But the potential to identify individuals that may lead on to future genetic discrimination will always remain: '(K)nowledge of a persons genetic makeup can be used to justify unequal treatment. For example, a candidate for a job may be excluded on the grounds of her genetic disposition to a future disease or a person wishing to buy health insurance could be refused on genetic grounds' (D'Abramo 2015: 1125). It is in this context that the 'right *not* to know' (in this case, one's genetic status) has been defended as a legitimate act to protect the autonomy and psychological status of individuals. This stands in contrast to the 'right to know' ethical principle recognised within international biomedical law, although the basis and conditions for the exercise of this right remain unclear in national legal frameworks. However, such a 'right not to know' has been criticised on the grounds that it contradicts a doctors' responsibility to inform patients in solidarity with family members. This is the situation that pertains when non-disclosure of some health risk factor could carry the potential of harm to a relative of that patient/donor who, without that vital information, could be deprived of preventive or therapeutic measures (Andorno 2004). The storing and long-term use of individual donated genomic data can therefore 'easily exacerbate the tension between individual rights and bioethical principles versus a population outlook and objectives of biobank research' (D'Abramo 2015: 1125).

Social studies of public attitudes towards the use of biobank data in research generally have shown high levels of trust and a positive vision of expected benefits. But examples of public mistrust over the uses of personal data and DNA samples are not exceptional. One of the well-known examples being the case of the US-owned deCODE Icelandic biobank. In 1996, the company planned to build a genomic database for the whole population of the island, intending to exploit the relatively homogeneous genomic profile of the Icelanders. However, the project ran into controversy as information gradually emerged about the lack of ownership and control that the population had over the commercialisation of their personal data. Many Icelanders found it completely unacceptable that their elected government had made a commercial deal with a private multinational company without any serious public consultation. This was a commercial deal that allowed access to their individual genetic information and medical records without their being any obvious health benefit to the population of Iceland as a whole.

Trust issues have also arisen in relation to unconsented use of biobank samples for the purposes of criminal forensic investigation. In such cases there is often a lack of ethical clarity when 'trading' between criminal databases and medical biobanks occurs. While all EU member states formally ban any speculative automated searches of biomedical databases for forensic purposes, in practice some countries have allowed this to occur. Equally, the use of national forensic criminal databases has from time-to-time raised concerns about the potential to abuse human rights and civil liberties. This stems from the fact that the individual data samples collated in forensic DNA databases are usually compulsorily obtained from individuals who have been arrested and accused of a crime, but not all those who have been accused are subsequently convicted. Forensic databases also collate DNA samples belonging to the victims of crime, as well to 'volunteers' (to refuse is to be labelled a suspect) in so-called 'DNA dragnets'. These have been termed 'warrantless searches' involving hundreds and even thousands of people who may be asked to provide blood or saliva with the aim of finding the person whose DNA was left at a crime scene (Machado and Silva 2015: 822).

Big Data Analytics and the Emergence of Bioinformatics

The notion of 'Big Data' has become a ubiquitous one over the course of the last decade. It refers to the existence of massive data sets that, because of their complexity and high degree of variability, cannot be analysed and interpreted by means of conventional statistical techniques. The term Big Data analytics' references the increasing computing processing power required to extract, manipulate, integrate, and store these data sets. The application of machine learning or artificial intelligence (AI) methodologies enables novel and potentially significant data patterns to be identified. This ability to harvest from a wide range of data sets is seen to offer particular opportunities for biomedical researchers to develop data-driven predictions complementary to knowledge-based hypothesis generation. At this point it important to bear in mind that such data is simply a collection of values existing in the form of characters, or numbers, or any simple quantities. If those values are not processed or analysed they have little or no meaning in and of themselves. Information is data that is processed so a human can read, understand, and use it, and processing data into information is the fundamental purpose of any computing system. Informatics is the systematic approach to the processing, representation, and communicating of information, and converting it into a practical form for scientists and policy-makers to effectively utilise.

The sources of Big Data of potential value for biomedicine are wide-ranging. These would include the personal and population-based biomedical data generated by primary and secondary care healthcare institutions, as well as being drawn from epidemiological research surveys, as well as data derived from laboratory-based research, including 'omics-based approaches such as genomics, proteomics, metabolomics, epigenomics, etc. These sources comprise individual medical records, population-level disease incidence and prevalence data sets, GWAS, experimental and literature reports, neuro and other clinical imaging data, as well as the many forms of sensor data. It would also include any type of individual or population-based data set that may not have obvious links to biomedicine, including data generated through social media use, online purchases, attitudinal surveys, and quantitative behavioural research of all types.

Genomics as a science was facing a significant crises of legitimation in the early 2000s, post-HGP. The volume, complexity, and variety of the genomic biodata that was being produced was compromised by the difficulties experienced in attempting to conceptualise, process, and analyse these vast quantities of material. The emergence of the interdisciplinary field of bioinformatics 'promised the solution to this problem through the imposition of order on the myriad uncertainties of the vast arrays of genomic data and, in so doing, provided a fresh legitimation and a new impetus to genomic science' (Salter and Salter 2017: 266). Bioinformatics began to change the ways of thinking about doing biomedical research. Certainly, by promoting the database-led approach of 'discovery science', bioinformatics has challenged the traditional paradigm of hypothesis-driven research (Salter and Salter 2017: 273). In building the connection between biology and information, the interdisciplinary power-balance of bioinformatics has arguably emphasised the mathematical over the biological. Bioinformatics has also challenged the ways in which biomedical science 'is organised and practiced through the forms of collaboration, division of labour and integrative strategies of models, data, theories, and software' (Salter and Salter 2017: 267). Writing from an ANT perspective, van Beren-Nawrocka et al. (2020) have argued that the paradigmatic approach of bioinformatics inevitably leads on to the 'enactment' of the human body as a calculable object. One whose characteristics and functioning 'can be calculated based on sequences alone' (2020: 92).

This rapid growth in the exploitation of Big Data has also raised significant privacy concerns, not least because it has preceded the establishment of effective national and international research ethics guidelines (de Mauro et al. 2016: 122). Over time as we have seen, the institutions of biomedical research became committed to the informed consent model, but given the sheer volume and variety of databases from which personal health information could now be extracted, ensuring individual consent for the use of this data has proved increasingly difficult. So that while in some cases, individuals might be re-contactable, 'it might still not be possible to inform them fully of the range of uses to which their data might be put by multiple users across countless ecosystems' (Xafis et al. 2019: 232). Big Data now opens up the potential to discover some hitherto unknown correlation between disease susceptibility and some other feature of the lives of individuals. But the danger of an over-reliance on Big Data in health science research is that those social and demographic groups who do not appear in proportional numbers in the range of social and other data sets that are drawn upon are then subsequently under-represented in that health research, 'thereby potentially exposing its members to harm or, at best, meaning that they miss out on benefits' (Xafis et al. 2019: 240). In response to these concerns, Xafis et al. (2019) have proposed an ethical framework that involves the application of three principles to cut across the decisions made about the appropriate use of Big Data in health science research. The first principle is 'respect for persons'. Meeting this requirement involves a willingness to engage with the public so as to understand and appreciate their concerns and expectations about the use of Big Data and to build public trust. The second principle is 'social license'. Meeting this principle means full disclosure to the public about the purpose of using Big Data in research activities in order to build 'positive public expectations associated with the perceived legitimacy of activities that have broad societal impacts'. The third principle is 'vulnerabilities and power'. This principle is concerned with raising self-awareness of the relative power that scientists and other Big

Data decision-makers have over the lives of others and should consider ways in which 'possible harms and wrongs may be mitigated or avoided entirely' (Xafis et al. 2019: 243).

At this point it is informative to examine a case study of the social and legal challenges that Big Data presents to regulatory frameworks designed to safeguard the use of personal data in biomedical research. The case study focuses on 'LifeGene', an ambitious Swedish national health and biobank project launched in 2010 and funded through a public-private partnership. 'LifeGene' represented a national strategic decision to utilise Big Data drawn from multiple data set sources across health and social welfare system domains in Sweden, on what was at the time an unprecedented scale. The project aimed to recruit 300,000 participants for the purpose of longitudinally collecting high-quality lifestyle and -omics data to facilitate large-scale prospective epidemiological research. Participants were asked to give their consent for the use and processing of personal lifestyle data collected specifically for this study, the storage of their blood and urine samples, and allow access to their personal health data from medical records and other health-relevant data drawn from Sweden's national registries; there were over 650 registered biobanks operating in 2019 (Biobank Sverige 2019). The longitudinal design of the project requires this data collection process to be repeated at five-year intervals over at least a period of twenty years. Individual data drawn from biological samples utilising 'omics technologies is aggregated into large data pools to identify biomarkers for the early detection of disease. But consistent with the bioinformatics methodology described above, rather than using traditional deductive techniques of theory building and development, algorithms are used to search for patterns and relationships 'that would be impossible to see without the aid of automated techniques i.e data-mining, machine-learning' (Cool 2015: 287).

Sweden is a country where historically there has been a close connection between the collection of national data to inform health and social welfare policies. Since 1947, all Swedish citizens and immigrants to the country have been assigned a 'personnummer' (an ID number) that they must use in all interactions with public institutions and even some commercial transactions. As a consequence, the data collected and stored by the Swedish government can easily be cross-linked with individual information held in other Swedish databases. In the past, this close tracking by the government of the health and social characteristics of its population was broadly acceptable to the public, there being a widespread trust in both the Swedish state and in the professionalism of scientists. But the LifeGene project is different in a number of ways from the previous uses of citizen data. Firstly, it is both a public *and* privately funded initiative, and secondly, the project is seeking to achieve lifelong sampling from participants, including children from birth. However, when public concerns were first raised with Sweden's Central Ethical Board about the programme, these two factors were not the primary concern, rather it was the fact that LifeGene was conceived as a big data resource rather than a stand-alone health research project.

The LifeGene biobank proposed collection of personal health and social data, in addition to individual biological samples meant it became subject to compliance with the Sweden's data protection laws. These laws stated that personal data can only be collected and stored for specified and authorised reasons, and not for unspecified general purposes (Cool 2015: 285). The Swedish Data Inspection Authority (DIA) therefore intervened to prevent LifeGene from processing digitalised personal data. In the public debate that followed, questions were raised about the legal protection for LifeGene participants and transparency in the use of their personal data. The response of the Swedish government in 2013 was to introduce a temporary legal change, specifically to allow LifeGene to resume personal data collection and so avoid the existing data protection legislation. The decision was made on the grounds that the biobanks project offered potentially significant health benefits for the country, both in terms of disease prevention and associated potential decrease in healthcare costs. This was a de facto recognition of the potential financial benefits associated with the commercial exploitation of the Big Data, which in effect outweighed the privacy concerns (Cool 2015: 287–290). As noted at the time in relation to this case, the biomedical research community can be a successful lobbyist when it is united, and when large investments have already been made and national pride is at stake (Asplund 2013).

As the European Commission have been slow to realise, the stakes involved in standardising European-wide data legislation able to protect the privacy of European citizens while allowing Big Data to flow freely across EU borders are high: 'For according to some estimates the value of European citizens' personal data has the potential to grow to nearly One Trillion Euro by 2020' (European Commission 2014—cited in Cool 2015: 291).

Conclusions: Limits to Governance

One major criticism of the framework of biomedical research regulation that has been established within the UK over the course of the last two decades is that it is not extensive enough! This is a viewpoint that sees only novelty not substance in the current governance arrangements for biomedical research. The short history of public-science engagement in the UK would be conceived as largely concerned to gain endorsement and legitimacy for pre-planned programmes of research science innovation. Rather than framing regulation in the narrow terms of what's 'good for science', a self-serving and arguably undemocratic approach, an alternative vision would require that a wider range of public voices be heard. Society as a whole has the right to expect tangible benefits from the biomedical sciences, not least because of the huge sums of public monies invested in research and development. It is also useful to be reminded that there are limits to science knowledge and prediction. Given the social, economic, and environmental uncertainties faced by society, biomedical science requires not only the trust of the public, but also the accountability mechanisms in place that can allow citizens to play a more active role in strategic decision-making, setting the priorities for the future direction of biomedical research.

Chapter Summary: Key Points

- *The 2004 Human Tissue Act rescinded the professional norms of discretion in the use of human tissue for research and established the principle of informed consent in law.*
- *Informed consent became the legal and ethical basis for the use of individual biological tissue in biomedical research in the UK.*
- *Human genome-editing research is now a global phenomenon, and its outcomes have the potential to impact all of humanity.*
- *Biobanks as repositories of personal and biological data have taken on a much more...*
- *...prominent role in facilitating biomedical research.*
- *The concept of 'biovalue' is used to highlight the actual contribution made by donors to research.*
- *The combining of personal health data with biomaterial has given rise to new legal and ethical challenges.*
- *There is an argument that there has been an over-reliance on the principle of informed consent to achieve respect for the autonomy and privacy of research participants.*
- *Not all information about research aims can be known at the time of donating personal biomaterial to biobanks that makes it difficult to fulfil the terms of informed consent.*
- *There is a difficulty in guaranteeing individual anonymity, when the potential of biobanks lies precisely in their ability to link biological to medical and other personalised data.*
- *Bioinformatics brings a mathematical and computational approach to biomedical science that some argue leads to the human body becoming merely a calculable object.*
- *Big Data analytics can result in an overly inductive process of 'letting the data speak for themselves', subsuming traditional deductive techniques of theory building.*
- *The potential financial benefits associated with the commercial exploitation of the Big Data can lead to a marginalisation of personal data privacy concerns.*

Bibliography

Andorno, R. (2004). The Right Not to Know: An Autonomy Based Approach. *Journal of Medical Ethics, 30*, 435–439.

Asplund, K. (2013, June). *Making an Illegal Big Data Study Legal. LifeGene: A Swedish Case Story*. Presentation at the National Ethics Committees Meeting. Dublin.

van Beren-Nawrocka, J., Consoli, L., & Zwart, H. (2020). Calculable Bodies: Analysing the Enactment of Bodies in Bioinformatics. *Biosocieties, 15*, 90–114.

Biobank Sverige. (2019). *Guide to Biobanks in Sweden.* Retrieved from www.biobanksverige.se.

Birch, K. (2012). Knowledge, Place and Power: Geographies of Value in the Bioeconomy. *New Genetics and Society, 31*(2), 183–201.

Braithwaite, J. (2013) The Regulatory State?. In E. Goodin (Ed.), *The Oxford Book of Political Science.* Oxford Books Online—Retrieved from https://www.oxfordhandbooks.com/.

Brownswood, R. (2010). Human Dignity, Biolaw and the Basis of Moral Community. *Journal international de bioethique, 21*(4), 21–40.

Campbell, A., McLean, S., Gutridge, K., & Harper, H. (2008). Human Tissue Legislation: Listening to the Professionals. *Journal of Medical Ethics, 34*(2), 104–108.

Cool, A. (2015). Detaching Data from the State: Biobanking and Building Big Data in Sweden. *Biosocieties, 11*(3), 277–295.

D'Abramo, F. (2015). Biobank Research, Informed Consent and Society. Towards a New Alliance? *Journal of Epidemiology and Community Health, 69*, 1125–1128.

De Mauro, A., Greco, M., & Grimaldi, M. (2016). A Formal Definition of Big Data Based on its Essential Features. *Library Review, 65*(3), 122–135.

Department of Health. (2005). *Review of the Human Fertilisation and Embryology Act: A Public Consultation*. London: DH.

European Commission. (2014). Progress on EU Data Protection Reform. EC MEMO/14/186.

Gillott, J. (2014). *Bioscience, Governance and Politics*. Basingstoke: Palgrave.

Gottweis, H., & Petersen, A. (Eds.). (2008). *Biobanks: Governance in Comparative Perspective*. London: Routledge.

Hansson, M. (2009). Ethics and Biobanks. *British Journal of Cancer, 100*(1), 8–12.

Health Research Authority. (2019). *The Use of Human Tissue in Research*. Retrieved from https://www.hra.nhs.uk/planning-and-improving-research/policies-standards-legislation/use-tissue-research/.

Hilgartner, S., Prainsack, B., & Hurlbut, B. (2017). Ethics as Governance in Genomics and Beyond. In U. Felt, R. Fouché, C. Miller, & L. Smith-Doerr (Eds.), *The Handbook of Science and Technology Studies* (4th ed., pp. 823–851). London, England: MIT Press.

Jasanoff, S. (2007). Technologies of Humility. *Nature, 450*(7166), 33.

Kaye, J., Moraia, L., Curren, L., Bell, J., Mitchell, C., Soini, S., et al. (2016). Consent for Biobanking: The Legal Frameworks of Countries in the BioSHaRE-EU Project. *Biopreservation and Biobanking, 14*(3), 195–200.

Kennedy, I. (2001). *The Report of the Public Inquiry into Children's Heart Surgery at the Bristol Royal Infirmary 1984–1995: Learning from Bristol-Cm 5207*. London: Department of Health.

Kristinsson, S. (2009). The Belmont Report's Misleading Conception of Autonomy. *AMA Journal of Ethics, 11*(8), 611–616.

Lander, E., Baylis, F., Zhang, F., Charpentier, E., & Berg, P. (2019). Adopt a Moratorium on Heritable Genome Editing. *Nature, 567*, 165–168.

Machado, H., & Silva, S. (2015). Public Participation in Genetic Databases: Crossing the Boundaries between Biobanks and Forensic DNA Databases through the Principle of Solidarity. *Journal of Medical Ethics, 41*, 820–824.

Meijer, I., Molas-Gallart, J., & Mattsson, P. (2012). Networked Research Infrastructures and Their Governance. The Case of Biobanking. *Science and Public Policy, 39*(4), 491–499.

Mitchell, R., & Waldby, C. (2010). National Biobanks, Clinical Labor, Risk Production, and the Creation of Biovalue. *Science, Technology and Human Values, 35*(3), 330–355.

O'Neill, O. (2003). Some Limits of Informed Consent. *Journal of Medical Ethics, 29*(1), 4–7.

Parliamentary Science and Technology Select Committee. (2018). *Genomics and Genome Editing in the NHS.* Retrieved from https://publications.parliament.uk/pa/cm201719/cmselect/cmsctech/349/34909.htm#_idTextAnchor050.

Price, D. (2009). *Human Tissue in Transplantation and Research.* Cambridge: Cambridge University Press.

Salter, B., & Salter, C. (2017). Controlling New Knowledge: Genomic Science, Governance and The Politics of Bioinformatics. *Social Studies of Science, 47*(2), 263–287.

Steinsbekk, K., Ursin, L., Skolbekkan, J., & Solberg, B. (2013). We're Not in it for the Money—Lay People's Moral Institutions on Commercial Use of 'Their' Biobank. *Medical Health Care and Philosophy, 16*, 151–162.

Strech, D. (2015). Ethical Review of Biobank Research: Should REC's Review Each Release of Material from Biobanks Operating under an Already Approved Broad Consent and Data Protection Model? *European Journal of Medical Genetics, 58*, 545–549.

Titmuss, R. (1970). *The Gift Relationship: From Human Blood to Social Policy*. Bristol: Policy Press.

Turner, A., Dallaire-Fortier, C., & Murtagh, M. (2013). Biobank Economics and the Commercialization Problem. *Spontaneous Generations, 7*(1), 69–80.

UK Biobank. (2019). *About UK Biobank*. Retrieved January 2020, from https://www.ukbiobank.ac.uk/about-biobank-uk/.

Xafis, V., Schaefer, G., Labude, M., Brassington, I., Ballingtyne, A., Lim, H., et al. (2019). An Ethics Framework for Big Data in Health and Research. *Asian Bioethics Review, 11*, 227–254.

Conclusion: Future Pathways in the Interdisciplinary Analysis of Biomedical Science

All the analytical material included within this textbook, the case studies, the ethnographic and social research, as well as the theoretical and philosophical discussions have been chosen to represent as broadly as possible, the constituents of an interdisciplinary approach to assessing the role now played by the biomedical sciences in contemporary society. This interdisciplinary approach is collectively termed Social Studies of Science and Technology (SSST).

Each of the chapters within the book has introduced examples of SSST research drawn from the disciplines of sociology, social policy, social psychology, political science, economics, and their sub-fields. The concern has been to achieve an analytical balance that reflects the wide scope of distinct disciplinary perspectives and methodological approaches applied to the study of science in society. The recognition of methodological difference at the level of epistemology *and* ontology is a reflection of the importance of acquiring an understanding and appreciation of the contribution of the philosophy of science.

From social constructionist analyses, we gain a critical insight into the 'cultures of knowing' that are drawn upon in laboratory work. Here the focus is on providing illustrative explanations of why the outputs of science cannot be value-free. This analysis highlights the uncertainties of science work and the practical necessity for biomedical scientists of achieving contingency in their research, sometimes at the expense of methodological consistency. And, as befits its origins in social anthropology, these STS approaches are primarily concerned with the cultural dynamics found with epistemic science communities, setting challenges to more idealised and uncritical accounts of biomedical science practice.

A critical realist-informed analyses draws attention to the ways in which social processes of interaction and construction serve to mediate the events occurring in the natural world. This is the view that human behaviour, whether individual or organisational, can never be conceptualised as purely an epiphenomenon of biological mechanisms. This is an approach characterised by an interdisciplinary reading of the processes of biosocial emergence as they arise from interactions occurring in the stratified (chemical, physical, biological, psychological, and social) open system that is the natural world.

I. Crinson, *The Biomedical Sciences in Society*,
https://doi.org/10.1007/978-981-15-9523-3

Many, if not most of those active in SSST research and analysis share a realist understanding of the materiality of the natural world in common with biomedical scientists. As such, SSST is often able to point to the ways in which biomedical science programmes of innovation are sometimes blind-sided to a set of realities that exist outside of their immediate scope of research concern. For example, unanticipated hazards and insecurities that can follow the single-minded pursuit of new biotechnological solutions, the unpredictability of the bio-social-environmental processes associated with epigenetic emergence, and an over-emphasis on seeking to identify a biological basis for human difference when it is our similarities that maybe more significant. Examples of these unanticipated outcomes, public trust issues, and the biases and reductionism that may be found in biomedical research practice have been discussed throughout the chapters of this book. The hope is that a mutual engagement can be established between biomedical science and SSST in assessing the interaction of the biological with the social. That is, an interdisciplinarity that can serve to support and inform the work of biomedical scientists in a rapidly changing world.

On a final note, this textbook was completed at the time the impact of the Covid-19 pandemic was making itself most strongly felt in the lives of us all. This global event has demonstrated, if we did not already know, the importance of adopting an interdisciplinary approach when managing public health responses, and in the building of the public consensus that is necessary for the implementation of the measures required to limit the social and economic fallout from such a devastating pandemic. Threats to the health of populations across the globe are only likely to be more frequent in future given the unpredictable outcomes of environmental degradation. Successful suppression of the global transmission of a virus necessitates robust predictive epidemiological modelling, credible public health interventions, and cutting edge virological research in the development of effective vaccines. But successful interventions also require a critical understanding of the cultural and economic context in which human interaction occurs and where global public trust in biomedical science is sustained or undermined. As such, the analytical field of SSST continues to make a positive critical contribution to the very necessary role undertaken by biomedical research science in safeguarding the future for our society.

Glossary

Acetylation Histone acetylation is a dynamic epigenetic modification that functions in the regulation of DNA-templated reactions, such as transcription, the first step in gene expression.

Bioassay Compares a test sample with an internationally applicable standard substance. In this case, the measurement of the pharmacological activity of new or chemically undefined substance.

Bright line A judicial rule utilised within the US legal framework that sets a basic standard to help resolve and clarify any ambiguity in law—when the need for a simple decision outweighs the need to weigh both sides of a particular issue.

Chromatin Is a complex of proteins called histones together with DNA: 147 base pairs of DNA wraps around the eight core histones to form the basic chromatin unit, the nucleosome. The function of chromatin is to efficiently package DNA into a small volume to fit into the nucleus of a cell and protect the DNA structure and sequence (NHGRI 2019)

Corticosterone One of the glucocorticoids, a hormone released in response to stress, secreted from the adrenal cortex; in humans, cortisol is the primary glucocorticoid. Both hormones exert their actions by binding to the glucocorticoid receptor (GR) present in almost all cells.

Domestic Division of Labour The ways in which care work and household responsibilities are divided between women and men within the family unit (extended or otherwise).

Ethnicity Within the social sciences, ethnicity is acknowledged as a social construction and used to denote some form of distinctive (i.e., from the majority population) set of cultural but not biological characteristics. These can include common geographical and ancestral origins, shared language, and various distinct traditions. These and other shared characteristics such as nationality, migrant status, and religion are frequently used as proxy measures for ethnic difference. Majority groups within a society can and frequently do impose the label of ethnic difference, but at the same time minority groups can themselves maintain these cultural boundaries. As such, ethnic difference is not fixed, but dynamic and changeable.

I. Crinson, *The Biomedical Sciences in Society*,
https://doi.org/10.1007/978-981-15-9523-3

Experimenters regress This refers to a loop of dependence between theory and evidence. In order to judge whether evidence is erroneous we must rely on theory-based expectations and to judge the value of competing theories we rely on evidence. Therefore, a circular relation exists between belief (or not) in an outcome and acceptance (or not) of the value of the apparatus producing it.

Gene chip technology Also known as DNA chip or biochip and it is a collection of microscopic DNA spots attached to a solid surface. This technique is used to measure the expression levels of large numbers of genes simultaneously or to genotype multiple regions of a genome. Each DNA spot contains a specific DNA sequence, known as 'probes'.

Genome editing Involves the application of technologies such as CRISPR to enable bioscientists to make changes to DNA, for example, to reduce risk of disease risk. The technologies that are utilised act like scissors, cutting the DNA at a specific spot, which can then be removed, added to, or replaced at the point where it was cut. The genome editing tool CRISPR was invented in 2009 and is more accurate, faster, and cheaper than older genome editing methods first used in research at the end of the 1990s.

Genome-wide association studies (GWAS) An examination of many common genetic variants in different individuals to see if any variant is associated with a known trait. GWAS typically focus on associations between single-nucleotide polymorphisms (SNPs) and traits for major diseases.

Genotype An individual's unique heritable genetic makeup. In genomics the term is also used to refer just to a particular gene or set of genes carried by an individual that influence the aspect of a phenotype (see below).

Gestalt theory Gestalt means 'configuration' or 'wholeness' and is a long-established approach within psychology that is concerned with how we perceive in a patterned way.

Haplotype A set of DNA variations, or polymorphisms, that tend to be inherited together. That is, a block of alleles at variants close together on just one chromosome occurring together more often than is expected by chance. A distinct haplogroup is one whose polymorphism variations have occurred over a period of more than 150,000 years and correlate with the geographic origins of identifiable populations traced through maternal lineage.

Hypothalamic pituitary adrenal (HPA) The neuro-hormonal system known as the HPA axis plays a ubiquitous role in the neurobiological central stress response system.

Imperfect markets In economic theory this refers to any economic market that does not meet the rigorous standards of a perfect competition, market equilibrium, and an unlimited number of buyers and sellers. An imperfect market is one in which individual buyers and sellers can influence prices and production, where there is no full disclosure of information about products and prices and where there are high barriers to entry or exit in the market.

Inscription devices Any item of apparatus or configuration able to transform a material substance into a usable representational form, such as a figure or diagram (e.g., the use of mass spectrometers in the pre-digital context of Latour and

Woolgar's study of laboratory work), or in recent times various computerised renderings of brain function through the use of colours representing increased blood flow.

Medicalisation Illich's (1976) thesis was a radical critique of biomedical science which asserted that more and more aspects of daily life had been brought into the medical sphere of influence, including those experiences that were once seen as a normal part of the human condition, such as pregnancy, childhood, ageing, and dying.

Methylation A mechanism that occurs by the addition of a methyl (CH_3) group to DNA that can lead to modification of the function of the genes and affect gene expression.

Moieties In organic chemistry this is a term used for part of a molecule.

Monoclonal antibody (MAB) Monospecific antibodies that are made by identical immune cells that are all clones of a unique parent B cell.

Off-label The use of pharmaceuticals for an unapproved indication or in an unapproved age group, dosage, or route of administration. Doctors in the UK can prescribe medications off-label. According to the GMC, off-label prescriptions must better serve patient needs than alternatives and must be supported by evidence or experience to demonstrate safety and efficacy.

Omics Refers to a field of study in biological sciences that ends with *-omics*, such as genomics, transcriptomics, proteomics, or metabolomics. Used as informal term to describe novel, comprehensive approaches for the analysis of *complete* genetic or molecular profiles of humans and other organisms. A global view on biological molecules such as DNA, RNA, proteins, and metabolites, in contrast to genetics, which focuses on *single* genes.

Ontological authority From the perspective of the philosophy of science, the ontological relates to the nature of being (discussed in detail in Chap. 2). However, within the natural sciences, the use of the term 'ontological authority' is more practical in that it relates to the overarching explanation of entities in a specific field of study, for example, genomics. It concerns the scientific authority to name, typologise, and conceptualise a given natural phenomenon.

Phenotype The visible or observable expression of the results of genes, combined with environmental influences. An organism's phenotype is determined by its genotype.

Plasmid A small, circular, double-stranded DNA molecule that replicates independently from the host's chromosomal DNA. They are mainly found in bacteria, but also exist naturally in archaea and eukaryotes such as yeast and plants.

Precision medicine This term has been utilised interchangeably with that of 'personalised medicine'. However, because of concerns that the term 'personalised' could be misinterpreted to imply that treatments and preventions were being uniquely developed for individuals, the term 'precision' came to be the preferred term. This was because it was seen to focus attention on identifying therapeutics that are effective for patients based on their precise genetic, environmental, and lifestyle factors.

Prospective cohort study A research study that follows groups of individuals who are alike in many ways (age) but may differ by certain characteristics (gender, ethnicity, social class, etc.) and compares them for a particular outcome over time. At the onset of the study, baseline data are collected on all the participants, so the risk of developing an outcome can be assessed.

Recombinant DNA (rDNA) DNA that has been created artificially. DNA from two or more sources is incorporated into a single recombinant (recombined) molecule.

Sexual dimorphism The condition where the two sexes of the same species exhibit different characteristics beyond the differences in their sexual organs.

Single nucleotide polymorphism (SNP) Each SNP represents a difference in a single DNA building block, called a nucleotide. For example, an SNP may replace the nucleotide cytosine (C) with the nucleotide thymine (T) in a certain stretch of DNA.

Somatic mutations An alteration in DNA that occurs after conception. Somatic mutations can occur in any of the cells of the body except the germ cells (sperm and egg) and therefore are not passed on to children. These alterations can, but do not always cause cancer or other diseases.

Stigma by association A sociological concept which describes the social process by which stigma affects not only people with physical or psychiatric disorders but their families as well, also referred to as 'courtesy' stigma (Goffman 1963).

Thyrotropin-releasing hormone (TRH) Its role in the human body is to act as the central regulator of the hypothalamic-pituitary-thyroid axis (HPT axis). The HPT axis plays a crucial role in regulating and maintaining somatic metabolism, thermogenesis, blood pressure, core body temperature, respiration rate, and food and water intake.

Transcriptional activation Genes contain the information needed to make functional molecules called proteins. The journey from gene to protein is complex and tightly controlled within each cell. It consists of two major steps: transcription and translation. Together, transcription and translation are known as gene expression. During the process of transcription, the information stored in a gene's DNA is transferred to a similar molecule called RNA (ribonucleic acid) in the cell nucleus.

Universal Health Care System As defined by the World Health Organisation, universal coverage means 'ensuring that all people have access to needed health services (including prevention, promotion, treatment, rehabilitation and palliation) of sufficient quality to be effective while also ensuring that the use of these services does not expose the user the financial hardship'.

Zoonotic Diseases A disease transmitted via harmful pathogens such as viruses, bacteria, fungi, and parasites, from animals to humans. The US Centre for Disease Control and Prevention has estimated that six out of every ten known infectious diseases in people can be spread from animals, and three out of every four new or emerging infectious diseases in people come from animals (CDC:2020). The link from BSE in cows to vCJD is discussed in Chap. 9, while the most recent devastating example of what is most likely to be a zoonotic disease is the Covid-19 pandemic.

Bibliography

Abi-Rached, J., & Rose, N. (2010). The Birth of the Neuromolecular Gaze. *History of the Human Sciences, 23*(1), 11–36.

Abi-Rached, J., Rose, N., & Mogoutov, A. (2010). *Mapping the Rise of the New Brain Sciences.* Working Paper BIOS no. 4. London. LSE.

Adolphs, R. (2003). Cognitive Neuroscience of Human Social Behavior. *Nature Reviews Neuroscience, 4*(3), 165–178.

Aharoni, E., Anderson, N., Barnes, J., Allen, C., & Kiehl, K. (2019). Mind the Gap: Toward an Integrative Science of the Brain and Crime. *BioSocieties, 14*, 463–468.

Ali-Khan, S., Krakowski, T., Tahir, R., & Daar, A. (2011). The Use of Race, Ethnicity and Ancestry in Human Genetic Research. *The HUGO (Human Genome Organisation) Journal, 5*, 47–63.

Allison, M. (2008). Is Personalized Medicine Finally Arriving? *Nature Biotechnology, 26*, 509–517.

Allmendinger, J. (2015) *Quests for Interdisciplinarity: A Challenge for the ERA and HORIZON 2020*—EUR 27370 EN. Brussels. European Commission.

American Psychiatric Association. (1987). *DSM-III: Diagnostic and Statistical Manual of Mental Disorders*. Washington, DC: APA.

American Psychiatric Association. (1994). *DSM-IV: Diagnostic and Statistical Manual of Mental Disorders*. Washington DC: APA.

American Psychiatric Association. (2013). *DSM-V: Diagnostic and Statistical Manual of Mental Disorder*. Washington, DC: APA.

Andorno, R. (2004). The Right Not to Know: An Autonomy Based Approach. *Journal of Medical Ethics, 30*, 435–439.

Apter, T. (2010). Delusions of Gender: The Real Science Behind Sex Differences by Cordelia Fine—Review. *Guardian*, 11 October 2010.

Asplund, K. (2013, June). *Making an Illegal Big Data Study Legal. LifeGene: A Swedish Case Story*. Presentation at the National Ethics Committees Meeting. Dublin.

Assaf, Y. (2018). New Dimensions for Brain Mapping. *Science, 362*(6418), 994–995.

Baghramian, M. (2013). Relativism about Science. In S. Psillos & M. Curd (Eds.), *The Routledge Companion to the Philosophy of Science* (2nd ed., pp. 268–179). London: Routledge.

Barad, K. (2007). *Meeting the Universe Halfway: Quantum Physics and the Entanglement of Matter and Meaning*. Durham, NC: Duke University Press.

Barnes, B., & Dupré, J. (2008). *Genomes and What to Make of Them*. London: University of Chicago Press.

Baron-Cohen, S. (2003). *The Essential Difference: Men, Women and the Extreme Male Brain*. London: Allen Lane.

Barry, A., & Born, G. (2013). Interdisciplinarity. In A. Barry & G. Born (Eds.), *Interdisciplinarity: Reconfigurations of the Social and Natural Sciences* (pp. 2–56). London: Routledge.

Bauer, M. (2009a). Editorial. *The Public Understanding of Science, 18*(4), 378–382.

I. Crinson, *The Biomedical Sciences in Society*,
https://doi.org/10.1007/978-981-15-9523-3

Bauer, M. (2009b). The Evolution of Public Understanding of Science—Discourse and Comparative Evidence. *Science, Technology and Society, 14*(2), 221–240.

Beauchamp, T., & Childress, J. (1979/2001). *Principles of Biomedical Ethics* (5th ed.). Oxford: Oxford University Press.

Beck, U. (1992). *Risk Society: Towards a New Modernity*. London: Sage.

Beck, U. (2006). *Living in the World Risk Society. A Hobhouse Memorial Public Lecture*. London: LSE.

van Beren-Nawrocka, J., Consoli, L., & Zwart, H. (2020). Calculable Bodies: Analysing the Enactment of Bodies in Bioinformatics. *Biosocieties, 15*, 90–114.

Berg, M. (1996). The Practices of Reading and Writing: The Constitutive Role of the Patient Record in Medical Work. *The Sociology of Health and Illness, 18*(4), 499–524.

Berger and Luckmann. (1967). *The Social Construction of Reality. A Treatise in the Sociology of Knowledge*. London: Allen Lane; The Penguin Press.

Bertorelli, T. (2016). Hope and Doubt in the Promise of Neuroimaging: The Case of Autism Spectrum Disorder. *Health, 20*(5), 505–522.

Bhaskar, R. (1978). *A Realist Theory of Science* (1st ed.). Hassocks: Harvester Press.

Bhaskar, R. (1989). *The Possibility of Naturalism: A Philosophical Critique of the Human Sciences*. Hassocks: Harvester Press.

Bhaskar, R. (1997). *A Realist Theory of Science* (2nd ed.). London: Verso Press.

Bhaskar, R., Danermark, B., & Price, L. (2018). *Interdisciplinarity and Wellbeing: A Critical Realist General Theory of Interdisciplinarity*. Abingdon: Routledge.

Biobank Sverige. (2019). *Guide to Biobanks in Sweden*. Retrieved from www.biobanksverige.se.

Birch, K. (2012). Knowledge, Place and Power: Geographies of Value in the Bioeconomy. *New Genetics and Society, 31*(2), 183–201.

Bleakley, A., & Bligh, J. (2009). Who Can Resist Foucault? *Journal of Medicine and Philosophy, 34*, 368–383.

Blickenstaff, J. (2005). Women and Science Careers: Leaky Pipeline or Gender Filter? *Gender and Education, 17*(4), 369–386.

Bloor, D. (1991). *Knowledge and Social Imagery* (2nd ed.). Chicago. University of Chicago Press (Original Version 1976: London. Routledge and Kegan Paul).

Bodmer Report. (1985). *The Public Understanding of Science*. London: The Royal Society. Retrieved September 2017, from https://royalsociety.org/~/media/Royal_Society_Content/policy/publications/1985/10700.pdf.

Borup, M., Brown, N., Konrad, K., & Van Lente, H. (2006). The Sociology of Expectations in Science and Technology. *Technological Analysis and Strategic Management, 18*(3), 285–298.

Bowlby, J. (1973). *Separation: Anger and Anxiety (Volume 2—Attachment and Loss)*. New York: Basic Books.

Braf, L., & Braf, D. (2013). The Neuropsychiatric Translational Revolution: Still Very Early and Still Very Challenging. *JAMA Psychiatry, 70*(8), 777–779.

Braithwaite, J. (2013) The Regulatory State?. In E. Goodin (Ed.), *The Oxford Book of Political Science*. Oxford Books Online—Retrieved from https://www.oxfordhandbooks.com/.

Broer, T., & Pickersgill, M. (2015). Targeting Brains, Producing Responsibilities: The Use of Neuroscience within British Social Policy. *Social Science and Medicine, 132*, 54–61.

Brosnan, C., & Michael, M. (2014). Enacting the 'Neuro' in Practice: Translational Research, Adhesion and the Promise of Porosity. *Social Studies of Science, 44*(5), 680–700.

Brown, A. (2002). Developing Realistic Philosophy. In A. Brown, S. Fleetwood, & J. Roberts (Eds.), *Critical Realism* (pp. 168–186). London: Routledge.

Brown, M. (2009). *Science in Democracy: Expertise, Institutions, and Representation*. Cambridge, MA: MIT Press.

Brownswood, R. (2010). Human Dignity, Biolaw and the Basis of Moral Community. *Journal international de bioethique, 21*(4), 21–40.

Bucchi, M., & Trench, B. (2016). Science Communication and Science in Society: A Conceptual Review in Ten Keywords. *Technoscienza, 7*(2), 151–168.

Burggren, W., Chapman, K., Keller, B., Monticino, M., & Torday, J. (2017). In R. Frodeman, J. Klein, & R. Pacheco (Eds.), *The Oxford Handbook of Interdisciplinarity* (2nd ed., pp. 101–113). Oxford: Oxford University Press.

Burnett, T. (2014) *What Is Scientism?* American Association for the Advancement of Science—Dialogue Science Ethics. Retrieved September 2019, from www.aaas.org/programs/dialogue-science-ethics-and-religion/what-scientism.

Cabinet Office. (2006). *Reaching Out: An Action Plan on Social Exclusion*. London: Cabinet Office.

Callard, F., & Fitzgerald, D. (2015). *Rethinking Interdisciplinarity across the Social Sciences and Neurosciences*. Basingstoke: Palgrave Macmillan.

Calvert, J., & Fujimura, J. (2011). Calculating Life? Duelling Discourses in Interdisciplinary Systems Biology. *Studies in History and Philosophy of Biological and Biomedical Sciences, 42*, 155–163.

Campbell, A., McLean, S., Gutridge, K., & Harper, H. (2008). Human Tissue Legislation: Listening to the Professionals. *Journal of Medical Ethics, 34*(2), 104–108.

Ceci, S., & Williams, W. (2011). Understanding the current causes of women's underrepresentation in science. *PNAS, 108*(8), 3157–3162.

Center for Cognitive Neuroscience. (n.d.). University of Pennsylvania. Retrieved September 2015, from http://ccn.upenn.edu.

Chao, H.-T., Liu, L., & Bellan, H. (2017). Building Dialogues between Clinical and Biomedical Research through Cross-Species Collaborations. *Seminars in Cell and Developmental Biology, 70*, 49–57.

Chen, S., Arsenault, C., Gingras, Y., & Larivière, V. (2015). Exploring the Interdisciplinary Evolution of a Discipline: The Case of Biochemistry and Molecular Biology. *Scientometrics, 102*, 1307–1323.

Cohen, S. (1972). *Folk Devils and Moral Panics*. London MacGibbon and Kee.

Cohen, S. (1999). Moral Panics and Folk Concepts. *Paedagogica Historica, 35*(3), 585–591.

Cohn, S. (2012). Disrupting Images: Neuroscientific Representations in the Lives in Psychiatric Patients. In S. Choudhury & J. Slaby (Eds.), *Critical Neuroscience: A Handbook of Social and Cultural Contexts of Neuroscience* (pp. 179–194). Chichester: Wiley Blackwell.

Collins, H. (2010). *Tacit and Explicit Knowledge*. Chicago: University of Chicago Press.

Collins, F. (2011). Reengineering Translational Science: The Time Is Right. *Science Translational Medicine, 3*(90).

Cool, A. (2015). Detaching Data from the State: Biobanking and Building Big Data in Sweden. *Biosocieties, 11*(3), 277–295.

Cooper, R., & Shallice, T. (2010). Cognitive Neuroscience: The Troubled Marriage of Cognitive Science and Neuroscience. *Topics in Cognitive Science, 2*, 398–406.

Coopmans, C., Vertesi, J., Lynch, M., & Woolgar, S. (2014). Introduction. In C. Coopmans, J. Vertesi, M. Lynch, & S. Woolgar (Eds.), *Representation in Scientific Practice Revisited* (pp. 1–12). Cambridge, MA: MIT Press.

Cope, W., & Kalantzis, M. (2009). Signs of Epistemic Disruption: Transformations in the Knowledge System of the Academic Journal. *First Monday, 14*(6).

Corporate Watch. (2005). *Newsletter*, 21. Retrieved from https://corporatewatch.org/content/newsletter-21-3-its-official-no-dark-machiavellian-conspiracy-new-nuclear-power.

Cousins, M., & Hussain, A. (1984). *Michel Foucault*. Basingstoke: Macmillan.

Coveney, C. (2011). Cognitive Enhancement? Exploring Modafinil Use in Social Context. In M. Pickergill & I. Van Keulan (Eds.), *Sociological Reflections on the Neurosciences* (pp. 203–228). Bingley: Emerald.

Creager, A. (2007). Introduction. In A. Creager, E. Lunbeck, & M. Norton Wise (Eds.), *Science without Laws: Model Systems, Cases, Exemplary Narratives* (pp. 1–20). Durham, NC: Duke University Press.

Crinson, I. (2004). The Politics of Regulation within the 'Modernised' NHS: The Case of Beta Interferon & the 'Cost-Effective' Treatment of Multiple Sclerosis. *Critical Social Policy, 24*(1), 30–49.

Cunliffe, V. (2015). Experience-Sensitive Epigenetic Mechanisms. Developmental Plasticity, and the Biological Embedding of Chronic Disease Risk. *Systems Biology and Medicine, 7*, 53–71.

D'Abramo, F. (2015). Biobank Research, Informed Consent and Society. Towards a New Alliance? *Journal of Epidemiology and Community Health, 69*, 1125–1128.
D'Argenio, V. (2018). The High-Throughput Analyses Era: Are We Ready for the Data Struggle? *High-Throughput, 7*(1), 8–10.
Danermark, B., Ekström, M., Jakobsen, L., & Karlsson, J. (2002). *Explaining Society: Critical Realism in the Social Sciences*. London: Routledge.
Daveney, J., Wang, S., Furbert-Harris, P., Apprey, V., Ittman, M., & Wang, B.-D. (2014). Genome-Wide Differentially Methylated Genes in Prostate Cancer Tissues from African-American and Caucasian Men. *Epigenetics, 10*(4), 310–328.
David, T., Gooch, K., Powell, S., & Abbott, L. (2003). *Birth to Three Matters: A Review of the Literature Compiled to Inform the Framework to Support Children in Their Earliest Years*. Department of Education and Skills—Research Report RR444. London: DfES Publications.
Davies, J. (2011). *Challenging Governance Theory*. Bristol: Policy Press.
De Mauro, A., Greco, M., & Grimaldi, M. (2016). A Formal Definition of Big Data Based on its Essential Features. *Library Review, 65*(3), 122–135.
De Rijcke, S., & Beaulieu, A. (2014). Networked Neuroscience: Brain Scans and Visual Knowing at the Intersection of Atlases and Databases. In C. Coopmans, J. Vertesi, M. Lynch, & S. Woolgar (Eds.), *Representation in Scientific Practice Revisited* (pp. 131–152). Cambridge, MA: MIT Press.
Denny, J., Rutter, J., Goldstein, D., Philippakis, A., Smoller, J., Jenkins, J., & Dishman, E. (2019). The 'All of US' Research Program. *The New England Journal of Medicine, 381*, 668–676.
Department of Business, Energy and Industrial Energy. (2018). *The Allocation of Funding for Research and Innovation*. London: BEIS.
Department of Education. (2019). *A-Level and Other 16–18 Results: 2018–19 (Revised): Maths and Science Tables*. Retrieved from https://www.gov.uk/government/organisations/department-for-education.
Department of Health. (2005). *Review of the Human Fertilisation and Embryology Act: A Public Consultation*. London: DH.
Deschauer, M. (2011). Black Box Brain: Anthropological Research on Neurosciences. In P. Gibas, K. Pauknerová, & M. Stella (Eds.), *Non-humans in Social Science: Animals, Spaces, Things*. Cˇervený Kostelec, Czech Rep. Pavel Mervart.
Doing, P. (2011). Tacit Knowledge. Discovery by or Topic for Science Studies? *Social Studies of Science, 41*(2), 301–306.
Dowie, J. (1999). Communication for Better Decisions: Not About 'Risk'. *Health, Risk & Society, 1*, 41–53.
Dowie, J. (2000). A Risky Decision: Managing without Risk. *Risk Management: An International Journal, 2*, 51–73.
Drolet, B., & Lorenzi, N. (2011). Translational Research: Understanding the Continuum from Bench to Bedside. *Translational Research, 157*(1), 1–6.
Dumit, J. (2003). *Picturing Personhood; Brain Scans and Biomedical Identity*. Princeton, NJ: Princeton University Press.
Dumit, J. (2012). *Drugs for Life: How Pharmaceutical Companies Define Our Health*. Durham & London: Duke University Press.
Dumit, J. (2014). How (Not) to Do Things with Brain Images. In C. Coopmans, J. Vertesi, M. Lynch, & S. Woolgar (Eds.), *Representation in Scientific Practice Revisited* (pp. 291–313). Cambridge, MA: MIT Press.
Duschauer, M. (2011). Black Box Brain. In P. Gibas, K. Pauknerova, & M. Stella (Eds.), *Non-humans in Social Science: Animals, Spaces, Things* (pp. 33–44). Prague: Pavel Mervart.
Duster, T. (2015). A Post-Genomic Surprise. The Molecular Re-inscription of Race in Science, Law and Medicine. *The British Journal of Sociology, 66*(1), 1–27.
Dyer, C. (2010). *Lancet* Retracts Wakefield's MMR Paper. *British Medical Journal, 340*, c396.
Ebrahim, S. (2012). Epigenetics, the Next Big Thing. *International Journal of Epidemiology, 41*(1), 1–3.
Education Policy Institute. (2019) *Analysis: A-Level Results Day 2019*. Retrieved December 2019, from https://epi.org.uk/publications-and-research/a-level-results-2019/.

Elliott, R., Camacho, E., Campbell, F., Jankovic, D., Martyn St James, M., Kaltenthaler, E., et al. (2018). *Prevalence and Economic Burden of Medication Errors in the NHS in England.* Sheffield. Policy Research Unit in Economic Evaluation of Health & Care Interventions (EEPRU).

Engdahl, E., & Lidskog, R. (2014). Risk, Communication and Trust: Towards an Emotional Understanding of Risk. *The Public Understanding of Science, 23*(6), 703–717.

Epstein, S. (2007). *Inclusion: The Politics of Difference in Medical Research.* Chicago: University of Chicago Press.

Erickson, M. (2016). *Science, Culture and Society* (2nd ed.). Cambridge: Polity Press.

European Bioinformatics Institute. (n.d.). *NHGRI—EBI GWAS Catalog.* Retrieved June 2020, from https://www.ebi.ac.uk/gwas/.

European Commission. (2009a). *Global Governance of Science—Report of the Expert Group on Global Governance of Science.* EUR 23616 EN. Luxembourg: Publications Office of the European Union.

European Commission. (2009b). *Gender Segregation in the Labour Market—Report of the Expert Group on Gender and Employment.* Luxembourg: Publications Office of the European Union.

European Commission. (2012). *Biobanks for Europe: A Challenge for Governance—Report of the Expert Group on Dealing with Ethical and Regulatory Challenges of International Biobank Research.* EUR 25302. Luxembourg: Publications Office of the European Union.

European Commission. (2014a). *Special Eurobarometer 419—Public Perceptions of Science, Research and Innovation.* Brussels: European Commission.

European Commission. (2014b). Progress on EU Data Protection Reform. EC MEMO/14/186.

European Commission. (2019). *She Figures 2018.* Brussels: European Commission.

European Commission. (2020). *EACEA National Policies Platform.* Retrieved February 2020, from https://eacea.ec.europa.eu/national-policies/.

European Medicines Agency. (n.d.). *EMA.* Retrieved September 2017, from http://www.ema.europa.eu/ema/.

European Union. (2014). *Horizon 2020 Programme (3.1.) Societal Challenges: Health, Demographic Change and Wellbeing.* Brussels: European Commission.

Fahr, K. and 20 Other Authors. (2015). Genetic and Epigenetic Fine-Mapping of Causal Autoimmune Disease Variants. *Nature, 518*(7539), 337–343.

FDA. (2011). *Guidance for Industry E16 Biomarkers Related to Drug or Biotechnology Product Development: Context, Structure, and Format of Qualification Submissions.* Silver Springs, MD: US Food and Drug Administration.

FDA. (2015). New Molecular Entity Approvals. Retrieved September 2015, from http://www.fda.gov/Drugs/DevelopmentApprovalProcess/DrugInnovation/ucm336115.htm.

FDA. (2019). Pharmacogenomic Drug Labeling. Retrieved November 2019, from www.fda.gov/drugs/science-and-research-drugs/table-pharmacogenomic-biomarkers-drug-labeling.

Fine, C. (2010). *Delusions of Gender.* London: Iconbooks.

Fishman, J., Mamo, L., & Grzanka, P. (2017). Sex, Gender and sexuality in Biomedicine. In U. Felt, R. Fouché, C. Miller, & L. Smith-Doerr (Eds.), *The Handbook of Science and Technology Studies* (4th ed., pp. 379–406). London, England: MIT Press.

Fitzgerald, D. (2014). The Trouble with Brain Imaging: Hope, Uncertainty and Ambivalence in the Neuroscience of Autism. *BioSocieties, 9*(3), 241–261.

Fitzgerald, D., & Callard, F. (2015). Social Science and Neuroscience Beyond Interdisciplinarity: Experimental Entanglements. *Theory, Culture & Society, 32*(1), 3–32.

Fleck, L. (1935/1979). *Genesis and the Development of a Scientific Fact.* Chicago: University of Chicago Press.

Fleetwood, S. (2013). *What Is (and What Isn't) Critical Realism.* Centre for Employment Studies Research (CSER) Seminar, 20th September 2013—University of the West of England.

Foresight Report. (2007). *Tackling Obesities—Future Choices.* London: UK Government Office for Science.

Foster, M., & Sharp, R. (2002). Race, Ethnicity, and Genomics: Social Classifications as Proxies of Biological Heterogeneity. *Genome Research, 12*, 844–850.

Foucault, M. (1967/1989). *Madness and Civilisation*. London: Routledge.

Foucault, M. (1973). *The Birth of the Clinic: An Archaeology of Medical Perception*. London: Tavistock Publications.

Franklin, T., et al. (2010). Epigenetic Transmission of the Impact of Early Stress across Generations. *Biological Psychiatry, 68*, 408–415.

van Frassen, B. (1980). *The Scientific Image*. Oxford: Clarendon Press.

Friese, C. (2013). Realizing Potential in Translational Medicine: The Uncanny Emergence of Care as Science. *Current Anthropology, 54*(S7), S129–S138.

Fuller, S. (2005). Is STS Truly revolutionary or merely Revolting? *Science & Technology Studies, 18*(1), 75–83.

Fumagalli, R. (2015). Five Theses on Neuroeconomics. *Journal of Economic Methodology, 23*(1), 77–96.

Gardner, J., Samuel, G., & Williams, C. (2015). Sociology of Low Expectations: Recalibration as Innovation Work in Biomedicine. *Science, Technology, & Human Values, 40*(6), 998–1021.

Gee, D. (2013). *More or Less Precaution? Late Lessons from Early Warnings: Science, Precaution, Innovation*. Copenhagen: European Environment Agency.

Gezelter, D. (2009). Being Scientific: Falsifiability, Verifiability, Empirical Tests, and Reproducibility. *The Open Science Project*. Retrieved September 2017, from http://openscience.org/.

Gibbons, S., & Kaye, J. (2007). Governing Genetic Databases: Collection, Storage and Use. *Kings Law Journal, 18*, 201–208.

Gillott, J. (2014). *Bioscience, Governance and Politics*. Basingstoke: Palgrave.

Gilman, S. (2010). The Art of Medicine: Moral Panic and Pandemics. *The Lancet, 375*, 1866–1867.

Ginsburg, G., & Philips, K. (2018). Precision Medicine from Science to Value. *Health Affairs, 37*(5), 694–701.

Goffman, E. (1963). *Stigma: Notes on the Management of Spoiled Identity*. Englewood Cliffs, NJ: Prentice-Hall.

Gottweis, H., & Petersen, A. (Eds.). (2008). *Biobanks: Governance in Comparative Perspective*. London: Routledge.

Gray, A. (2004). Governing Medicine: An Introduction. In A. Gray & S. Harrison (Eds.), *Governing Medicine: Theory and Practice* (pp. 5–20). Maidnhead: Open University Press.

Green, J. (2009). Is It Time for the Sociology of Health to Abandon 'Risk'? *Health, Risk and Society, 11*(6), 493–508.

Greenfield, A. (2017). *Radical Technologies: The Design of Everyday Life*. London: Verso.

Gregory, J. (2001). Public Understanding of Science: Lessons from the UK Experience. *SciDevnet*. Retrieved September 2016, from http://www.scidev.net/global/communication/feature/public-understanding-of-science-lessons-from-the.html.

Griffiths, P., & Stotz, K. (2013). *Genetics and Philosophy*. Cambridge: Cambridge University Press.

Gunn, G. (1992). Interdisciplinary Studies. In J. Gibaldi (Ed.), *Introduction to Scholarship in Modern Languages and Literatures* (pp. 239–161). New York: Modern Language Association of America.

Hacking, I. (1983). *Representing and Intervening: Introducing Topics in the Philosophy of Natural Science*. Cambridge: Cambridge University Press.

Hagner, M. (2012). Perception, Knowledge and Freedom in the Age of Extremes: On the Historical Epistemology of Ludwik Fleck and Michael Polanyi. *Studies in Eastern European Thought, 12*(64), 107–120.

Handy, D., Castro, R., & Loscalazo, J. (2011). Epigenetic Modifications: Basic Mechanisms and Role in Cardiovascular Disease. *Circulation, 123*(19), 2145–2156.

Hansson, M. (2009). Ethics and Biobanks. *British Journal of Cancer, 100*(1), 8–12.

Haraway, D. (1985). *A Cyborg Manifesto: Science , Technology, and Socialist—Feminism in the late Twentieth Century*. Minneapolis: University of Minnesota Press.

Harrington, J., & Hauskeller, C. (2014). Translational Research: An Imperative Shaping the Spaces in Biomedicine. *Technoscienza, 5*(1), 191–201.

Harrison, B., & Pentalis, C. (2010). Cognitive Subtraction. In I. Stolerman (Ed.), *Encyclopaedia of Psychopharmacology*. Berlin: Springer.

Harrison, G., & Ross, D. (2012). The Methodologies of Neuroeconomics. In C. Marchionni & J. Vromen (Eds.), *Neuroeconomics: Hype or Hope?* (pp. 85–96). London: Routledge.

Haseltine, W. (1998). Not Quite Pharmacogenomics. *Nature Biotechnology, 16*, 1295–1296.

Healey, M., & Hodgkinson, G. (2014). Rethinking the Philosophical and Theoretical Foundations of Organizational Neuroscience: A Critical Realist Alternative. *Human Relations, 67*(7), 765–792.

Health Research Authority. (2019). *The Use of Human Tissue in Research*. Retrieved from https://www.hra.nhs.uk/planning-and-improving-research/policies-standards-legislation/use-tissue-research/.

Hedgecoe, A., & Martin, P. (2003). The Drugs Don't Work: Expectations and the Shaping of Pharmacogenetics. *Social Studies of Science, 33*, 327–364.

Heijmans, B., Tobi, E., & Stein, E. (2008). Persistent Epigenetic Differences Associated with Prenatal Exposure to Famine in Humans. *Proceedings of the National Academy of Sciences, 105*, 17046–17049.

Hickok, G. (2014). *The Myth of Mirror Neurons: The Real Neuroscience of Communication and Cognition*. Norton.

Higher Education Statistics Agency. (2019). *What Do HE Students Study?* Retrieved from https://www.hesa.ac.uk/data-and-analysis/students/what-study.

Hilgartner, S., Prainsack, B., & Hurlbut, B. (2017). Ethics as Governance in Genomics and Beyond. In U. Felt, R. Fouché, C. Miller, & L. Smith-Doerr (Eds.), *The Handbook of Science and Technology Studies* (4th ed., pp. 823–851). London, England: MIT Press.

Horgan, J. (2019, August 5). We Should All Be Science Critics. *Scientific American*. Retrieved from https://blogs.scientificamerican.com/cross-check/we-should-all-be-science-critics/.

Horrobin, D. (2003). Modern Biomedical Research: An Internally Self-Consistent Universe with Little Contact with Medical Reality? *Nature Reviews: Drug Discovery, 2*, 151–154.

House of Commons Science and Technology Select Committee. (2014). Women in Scientific Careers—Sixth Report of Session 2013–14. HC 701. http://www.publications.parliament.uk/pa/cm201314/cmselect/cmsctech/701/701.pdf.

House of Lords. (2000). Select Committee on Science and Technology, Third Report—*Science and Society*. Retrieved from http://www.publications.parliament.uk/pa/ld199900/ldselect/ldsctech/38/3801.htm.

Hughes, R. (2011). Are the Predictors of Women's Persistence in STEM Painting the Full Picture? *Gender, Science and Technology, 3*(3), 547–570.

Hyman, S. (2008). A Glimmer of Light for Neuropsychiatric Disorders. *Nature, 455*(7215), 890–893.

Irwin, A. (2008). STS Perspectives on Scientific Governance. In E. J. Hackett, O. Amsterdamska, M. Lynch, & J. Wajcman (Eds.), *The Handbook of Science and Technology Studies* (3rd ed., pp. 583–607). Cambridge, MA: MIT Press.

Irwin, A., & Wynne, B. (1996). *Misunderstanding Science? The Public Reconstruction of Science and Technology*. Cambridge: Cambridge University Press.

ISOGG - International Society of Genetic Genealogy. (2019). List of Testing Companies. isogg.org/wiki/List_of_DNA_testing_companies – accessed December 2019.

Jacobs, S. (2006). Models of Scientific Community. *Interdisciplinary Science Reviews, 31*(2), 163–173.

Jantsch, E. (1970/1972). Inter- and Transdisciplinary University: A Systems Approach to Education and Innovation. *Higher Education, 1*, 7–37.

Jasanoff, S. (2007). Technologies of Humility. *Nature, 450*(7166), 33.

Jasanoff, S. (2016). The Floating Ampersand: STS Past and STS to Come. *Engaging Science, Technology, and Society, 2*, 227–237.

Jasienska, G. (2009). Low Birth Weight of Contemporary African Americans: An Intergenerational Effect of Slavery? *American Journal of Human Biology, 21*, 6–24.

Jassanoff, S. (2013). Fields and Fallows: A Political History of STS. In A. Barry & G. Born (Eds.), *Interdisciplinarity: Reconfigurations of the Social and Natural Sciences* (pp. 99–118). London: Routledge.

Jay, V. (2000). The Legacy of Jean-Martin Charcot. *Archives of Pathology & Laboratory Medicine, 124*(1), 10–11.

Joel, D., et al. (2015). Sex Beyond the Genitalia: The Human Brain mosaic. *Proceedings of the National Academy of Sciences of the USA, 112*(50), 15468–15473.

Jones, R., & Wilsdon, J. (2018). *The Biomedical Bubble: Why UK Research and Innovation Needs a Greater Diversity of Priorities, Politics, Places and People*. London: NESTA.

Jordan-Young, R. (2011). *Brainstorm: The Flaws in the Science of Sex Difference*. Cambridge, MA: Harvard University Press.

Kagan, J. (1998). *Three Seductive Ideas*. Harvard, MA: Harvard University Press.

Kastenhofer, K. (2013). Two Sides of the Same Coin? The (Techno)epistemic Cultures of Systems and Synthetic Biology. *Studies in History and Philosophy of Biological and Biomedical Sciences, 44*, 130–140.

Kaye, J., Moraia, L., Curren, L., Bell, J., Mitchell, C., Soini, S., et al. (2016). Consent for Biobanking: The Legal Frameworks of Countries in the BioSHaRE-EU Project. *Biopreservation and Biobanking, 14*(3), 195–200.

Keating, P., & Cambrosio, A. (2003). *Biomedical Platforms: Realigning the Normal and Pathological in Late-Twentieth Century Medicine*. Cambridge, MA: MIT Press.

Kennedy, I. (2001). *The Report of the Public Inquiry into Children's Heart Surgery at the Bristol Royal Infirmary 1984–1995: Learning from Bristol-Cm 5207*. London: Department of Health.

Kessler, R., Bergland, P., & Demler, O. (2005). Lifetime Prevalence and Age-of-Onset Distributions of DSM-IV Disorders in the National Comorbidity Survey Replication. *Archives of General Psychiatry, 62*(6), 593–602.

Kitano, H. (2004). Biological Robustness. *Nature Review Genetics, 59*, 826–837.

Klein, J. (2010). Taxologies of Interdisciplinarity. In R. Frodeman, J. Klein, & R. Pacheco (Eds.), *The Oxford Handbook of Interdisciplinarity* (1st ed., pp. 15–30). Oxford: Oxford University Press.

Klein, J. (2017). Typologies of Interdisciplinarity. In R. Frodeman, J. Klein, & R. Pacheco (Eds.), *The Oxford Handbook of Interdisciplinarity* (2nd ed., pp. 21–35). Oxford: Oxford University Press.

Knorr Cetina, K. (1981). *The Manufacture of Knowledge: An essay on the Constructivist and Contextual Nature of Science*. Oxford: Pergamon Press.

Knorr Cetina, K. (1983). The Ethnographic Study of Scientific Work: Towards a Constructionist Interpretation of Science. In K. Knorr Cetina & M. Mulkay (Eds.), *Science Observed: Perspectives on the Social Study of Science* (pp. 125–140). London: Sage.

Knorr Cetina, K. (1999). *Epistemic Cultures: The Cultures of Knowledge Societies*. Cambridge, MA: Harvard University Press.

Knorr Cetina, K. (2005). Culture in Global Knowledge Societies: Knowledge Cultures and Epistemic Cultures. In S. Jacobs & N. Weiss Hanrahan (Eds.), *The Blackwell Companion to the Sociology of Culture* (pp. 65–79). Oxford: Blackwell.

Kohler, R. (1982). *From Medical Chemistry to Biochemistry; The Making of a Biomedical Discipline*. Cambridge: Cambridge University Press.

Kolb, B., & Gibb, R. (2011). Brain Plasticity and Behaviour in the Developing Brain. *Journal of the Canadian Academy of Child and Adolescent Psychiatry, 20*(4), 265–276.

Krakauer, J., Ghazanfar, A., Gomez-Marin, A., MacIver, M., & Poeppel, P. (2017). Neuroscience Needs Behavior: Correcting a Reductionist Bias. *Neuron, 93*, 480–490.

Krautwurst, U. (2014). *Culturing Bioscience*. Toronto: University of Toronto Press.

Krebs, K., & Milani, L. (2019). Translating Pharmacogenomics into Clinical Decisions: Do Not Let the Perfect Be the Enemy of the Good. *Human Genomics, 13*, 39.

Kristinsson, S. (2009). The Belmont Report's Misleading Conception of Autonomy. *AMA Journal of Ethics, 11*(8), 611–616.

Kuhn, T. (1970). *The Structure of Scientific Revolutions* (2nd ed.). Chicago: Chicago University Press.

Kumaraswamy, N. C., et al. (2019). Race Specific Alterations in DNA Methylation Among Middle-Aged African American and Whites with Metabolic Syndrome. *Epigenetics, 14*. https://doi.org/10.1080/15592294.2019.1695340.

Kuzawa, C., & Sweet, E. (2009). Epigenetics and the Embodiment of Race: Developmental Origins of US Racial Disparities in Cardiovascular Health. *American Journal of Human Biology, 21*, 2–15.

Kyte, S., & Riegle-Crumb, C. (2017). Perceptions of the Social Relevance of Science: Exploring the Implications for Gendered Patterns in Expectations of Majoring in STEM Fields. *Social Sciences, 6*(19), 1–13.

van der Laan, A., & Boenink, M. (2015). Beyond Bench and Bedside: Disentangling the Concept of Translational Research. *Health Care Analysis, 23*, 32–49.

Landecker, H. (2007). *Culturing Life*. London: Harvard University Press.

Lander, E., Baylis, F., Zhang, F., Charpentier, E., & Berg, P. (2019). Adopt a Moratorium on Heritable Genome Editing. *Nature, 567*, 165–168.

Lappé, M. (2018). The Paradox of Care in Behavioral Epigenetics: Constructing Early Life Adversity in the Lab. *BioSocieties, 13*(4), 698–714.

Lappé, M., & Landecker, H. (2015). How the Genome Got a Life Span. *New Genetics and Society, 34*(2), 152–176.

Latour, B. (1987). *Science in Action: How to Follow Scientists and Engineers through Society*. Cambridge, MA: Harvard University Press.

Latour, B. (1988). The Politics of Explanation: An Alternative. In S. Woolgar (Ed.), *Knowledge and Reflexivity: New Frontiers in the Sociology of Knowledge* (pp. 155–176). London: Sage.

Latour, B. (1990). On Actor-Network Theory. A Few Clarifications Plus More Than a Few Complications. *Philosophie, 25*(3), 47–64.

Latour, B. (1999). *Pandora's Hope: Essays on the Reality of Science Studies*. Cambridge, MA: Harvard University Press.

Latour, B. (2005). *Reassembling the Social: An Introduction to Actor-Network-Theory*. Oxford: Oxford University Press.

Latour, B., & Woolgar, S. (1979). *Laboratory Life: The Construction of Scientific Facts*. Princeton, NJ: Princeton University Press.

Law, J. (1992). *Notes on the Theory of the Actor Network: Ordering, Strategy and Heterogeneity*. Centre for Science Studies, Lancaster University, Lancaster.

Law, J. (2002). *Aircraft Stories: Decentering the Object in Technoscience*. Durham, NC and London: Duke University Press.

Legrenzi, P. & Umiltà, C. (2011). Neuromania: *On the Limits of Brain Science*. Oxford. Oxford University Press.

Levin, N. (2014). What's Being Translated in Translational Research? *Technoscienza, 5*(1), 91–113.

Lewens, T. (2015). *The Meaning of Science*. London: Pelican Books.

Linder, A., & Svedberg, W. (2019). Review of Average Sized Male and Female Occupant Models in European Regulatory Safety Assessment Tests and European Laws: Gaps and Bridging Suggestions. *Accident Analysis and Prevention, 127*, 156–162.

Lipinski, K., Barber, L., Davies, M., Ashenden, M., Sottoriva, A., & Gerlinger, M. (2016). Cancer Evolution and the Limits of Predictability in Precision Cancer Medicine. *Trends in Cancer, 2*(1), 49–63.

Lloyd, S., & Müller, R. (2018). Situating the Biosocial: Empirical Engagements with Environmental Epigenetics from the Lab to the Clinic. *BioSocieties, 13*(4), 675–680.

Lock, M. (2015). Comprehending the Body in the Era of the Epigenome. *Current Anthropology, 56*(2), 151–117.

Locke, J. (1689/1975). An Essay Concerning Human Understanding. In P. Nidditch (Ed.), Oxford: Oxford University Press.

Lowe, P., Lee, E., & Macvarish, J. (2015). Biologising Parenting: Neuroscience Discourse, English Social and Public Health Policy and Understandings of the Child. *Sociology of Health and Illness, 37*(2), 198–211.

Luhmann, N. (1979). *Trust and Power*. Chichester: Wiley.

Luhmann, N. (2000). Familiarity, Confidence, Trust: Problems and Alternatives. In G. Diego (Ed.), *Trust: Making and Breaking Cooperative Relations*. Oxford: University of Oxford.

Lumey, L., Stein, A., Kahn, H., Van der Pal de Bruin, K., Blauw, G., Zybert, P., & Susser, E. (2007). Cohort Profile: The Dutch Hunger Winter Families Study. *International Journal of Epidemiology, 36*(6), 1196–1204.

Lyall, C., Papiaoannou, T., & Smith, J. (2009). Governance in Action in the Life Sciences: Some Lessons for Policy. In C. Lyall, T. Papiannou, & J. Smith (Eds.), *The Limits to Governance: The Challenge of Policy-Making for the New Life Sciences* (pp. 250–271). Aldershot: Ashgate.

Lynch, M. (1985). *Art and Artefact in Laboratory Science*. London: Routledge.

Machado, H., & Silva, S. (2015). Public Participation in Genetic Databases: Crossing the Boundaries between Biobanks and Forensic DNA Databases through the Principle of Solidarity. *Journal of Medical Ethics, 41*, 820–824.

Madison, G., & Fahlman, P. (2020). Sex Differences in the Number of Scientific Publications and Citations When Attaining the Rank of Professor in Sweden. *Studies in Higher Education* (Online Version Only—February 2020).

Maglo, K. (2010). Genomics and the Conundrum of Race: Some Epistemic and Ethical Considerations. *Perspectives in Biology and Medicine, 53*(3), 357–372.

Mäki, U. (2016). Philosophy of Interdisciplinarity. What? Why? How? *European Journal of the Philosophy of Science, 6*, 327–342.

Malik, K. (2019). Einstein Got It Right—Philosophy and Science Do Go Hand in Hand. *The Guardian*, 24 February 2019.

Marchionni, C., & Vromen, J. (2012). Introduction. In C. Marchionni & J. Vromen (Eds.), *Neuroeconomics: Hype or Hope?* (pp. 1–7). London: Routledge.

Marante, D. (2020). Science and Technology Studies and Its Interdisciplinarity Problem. *Areo magazine.com*, 23 July 2020.

Martin, P., Brown, N., Coveney, C., & Williams, S. (2011). Pharmaceutical Cognitive Enhancement: Interrogating the Ethics, Addressing the Issues. In I. Segev & H. Markham (Eds.), *Augmenting Cognition* (pp. 179–192). Lausanne: EPFL Press.

Mayer-Schönberger, V., & Cukier, K. (2013). *Big Data: A Revolution That Will Transform How We Live, Work and Think*. London: John Murray.

Meijer, I., Molas-Gallart, J., & Mattsson, P. (2012). Networked Research Infrastructures and Their Governance. The Case of Biobanking. *Science and Public Policy, 39*(4), 491–499.

Melhuish, E., Gardiner, J., & Morris, S. (2017). *Study of Early Education and Development (SEED): Impact Study on Early Education Use and Child Outcomes up to Age Three*. London: DfES Publications.

Meloni, M. (2014). How Biology Became Social, and What It Means for Social Theory. *The Sociological Review, 62*(3), 593–614.

Meloni, M. (2017). Race in an Epigenetic Time: Thinking Biology in the Plural. *The British Journal of Sociology, 68*(3), 389–409.

Meloni, M., & Testa, G. (2014). Scrutinizing the Epigenetics Revolution. *Biosocieties, 9*(4), 431–456.

Meloni, M., Williams, S., & Martin, P. (2016). The Biosocial: Sociological Themes and Issues. In M. Meloni, S. Williams, & P. Martin (Eds.), *Biosocial Matters: Rethinking Sociology-Biology Relations in the Twenty-First Century* (pp. 7–25). Chichester: John Wiley & Sons.

Meynan, G. (2016). Neurolaw: Recognizing Opportunities and Challenges for Psychiatry. *Journal of Psychiatry and Neuroscience, 41*(1), 3–5.

Miller, G. (2003). The Cognitive Revolution: A Historical Perspective. *Trends in Cognitive Science, 7*(3) 141–144.

Mitchell, R., & Waldby, C. (2010). National Biobanks, Clinical Labor, Risk Production, and the Creation of Biovalue. *Science, Technology and Human Values, 35*(3), 330–355.

Mogil, J. (2009). Animal Models of Pain: Progress and Challenges. *Nature Reviews—Neuroscience, 10*, 283–294.

Mol, A.-M., & Law, J. (2006). Complexities: An introduction. In J. Law & A.-M. Mol (Eds.), *Complexities: Social Studies of Knowledge Practices* (pp. 1–22). Durham, NC: Duke University Press.

Monsinger-Reif, A., Jorgenson, E., Relling, M., Kroetz, D., Weinshilboum, R., Cox, N. J., & Roden, D. (2013). Genome-Wide Association Studies in Pharmacogenomics: Successes and Lessons. *Pharmacogenet Genomics, 23*(8), 383–394.

Moran, M. (2003). *The British Regulatory State*. Cambridge: Cambridge University Press.

Morrison, D., & Grzanka, P. (2017). Postracial Fantasies and the Reproduction of Scientific Racism. *Communication and Sociology, 2*.

Müller, C., & Schumann, G. (2011). To Use or Not to Use: Expanding the View on Non-Addictive Psychoactive Drug Consumption and Its Implications. *Behavioral and Brain Sciences, 34*, 328–347.

Müller, R., Hanson, C., & 20 Other Authors. (2017). The Biosocial Genome? *EMBO Reports, 19*(10), 1677–1682.

Nadal, M., & Skov, M. (2015). Neuroesthetics. In J. Wright (Ed.), *International Encyclopedia of the Social & Behavioral Sciences* (2nd ed., pp. 656–663). Elsevier.

National Academy of Sciences, National Academy of Engineering, and Institute of Medicine. (2005). *Facilitating Interdisciplinary Research*. Washington, DC: National Academies Press.

National Commission for the Protection of Human Subjects of Biomedical and Behavioral Research. (n.d.). *The Belmont Report: Ethical Principles and Guidelines for the Protection of Human Subjects of Research*. Bethesda, MD: US Government Printing Office.

National Human Genome Research Institute (NHGRI). (n.d.). Retrieved November 2019, from https://www.genome.gov/about-genomics/.

National Institutes of Health (NIH). (n.d.-a). *What Are Single Nucleotide Polymorphisms (SNPs)?* Retrieved November 2019, from https://ghr.nlm.nih.gov/primer/genomicresearch/snp.

National Institutes of Health (NIH). (n.d.-b). *What Is Epigenetics?* Retrieved January 2020, from https://ghr.nlm.nih.gov/primer/howgeneswork/epigenome.

Naughton, J. (2012). Thomas Kuhn: The Man Who Changed the Way the World Looked at Science. *Guardian*, 19 August 2012.

Newton, T. (2016). The Turn to Biology. In M. Meloni, S. Williams, & P. Martin (Eds.), *Biosocial Matters: Rethinking Sociology-Biology Relations in the Twenty-First Century* (pp. 117–133).

NHS. (2017). Retrieved May 2019, from www.nhs.uk/news/neurology/could-brain-scans-be-used-to-screen-for-autism/.

NHS. (2018). Genomics Education Programme. Retrieved September 2019, from www.genomicseducation.hee.nhs.uk.

NHS. (2019). *Childhood Vaccination Coverage Statistics—England: 2019–20*. https://digital.nhs.uk/data-and-information/publications/statistical/nhs-immunisationstatistics/england---2019-20.

Norris, C. (2014). What Strong Sociologists Can Learn from Critical Realism: Bloor on the History of Aerodynamics. *Journal of Critical Realism, 13*(1), 3–37.

O'Neill, O. (2003). Some Limits of Informed Consent. *Journal of Medical Ethics, 29*(1), 4–7.

Olson, S. (2002). *Mapping Human History*. Houghton: Mifflin Books.

Orman, R. (2016). 'Paradigm' as a Central Concept in Thomas Kuhn's Thought. *International Journal of Humanities and Social Science, 6*(10), 47–52.

Osbourne, T. (2013). Inter That Discipline! In A. Barry & G. Born (Eds.), *Interdisciplinarity: Reconfigurations of the Social and Natural Sciences* (pp. 82–98). London: Routledge.

Palsson, G. (2016). Unstable Bodies: Biosocial Perspectives on Human Variation. In M. Meloni, S. Williams, & P. Martin (Eds.), *Biosocial Matters: Rethinking Sociology-Biology Relations in the Twenty-First Century* (pp. 100–116).

Parliamentary Science and Technology Select Committee. (2018). *Genomics and Genome Editing in the NHS*. Retrieved from https://publications.parliament.uk/pa/cm201719/cmselect/cmsctech/349/34909.htm#_idTextAnchor050.

Patterson, M., & Johnson, J. (2012). Theorizing the Obesity Epidemic: Health Crisis, Moral Panic and Emerging Hybrids. *Social Theory & Health, 10*, 265–291.

Peltonen, L., & McKusick, V. (2001). Dissecting Human Disease in the Postgenomic Era. *Science, 291*(5507), 1224–1229.

Perez, M., & Lehner, B. (2019). Intergenerational and Transgenerational Epigenetic Inheritance in Animals. *Nature Cell Biology, 21*(2), 143–159.

Perez-Rodriguez, J., & de la Fuente, A. (2017). Now is the Time for a Postracial Medicine: Biomedical Research, the National Institutes of Health, and the Perpetuation of Scientific Racism. *American Journal of Bioethics, 17*(9), 36–47.

Philips, N. L. (2000). *The BSE inquiry. Volume 1, Findings and Conclusions*. London: Stationary Office.

Pickersgill, M. (2013). The Social Life of the Brain: Neuroscience in Society. *Current Sociology, 61*(3), 322–340.

Pickersgill, M., & Van Keulan, I. (Eds.). (2012). *Sociological Reflections on the Neurosciences*. Emerald: Bingley.

Pilgrim, D. (2019). Mental Health, Subjectivities and Forms of Neuroscience: A Critical Realist Examination. *Social Theory and Health., 17*, 140–157.

Piller, F., & Tseng, M. (2010). *Handbook of Research in Mass Customization and Personalization*. New Jersey: World Scientific Books.

Pinel, C., Prainsack, B., & McKevitt, C. (2018). Markers as Mediators: A Review and Synthesis of Epigenetics Literature. *Biosocieties, 13*(1), 276–303.

Polanyi, M. (1958). *Personal Knowledge: Towards a Post-Critical Philosophy*. Chicago: Chicago University Press.

Polanyi, M. (1985). *Implizites Wissen [1966]*. Frankfurt am Main: Suhrkamp.

Political Science Association—PSA. (2019). Why Do UK Universities Have Such Large Gender Pay Gaps? Retrieved December 2019, from https://www.psa.ac.uk/psa/news/why-do-uk-universities-have-such-large-gender-pay-gaps.

Popper, K. (1963). *Conjectures and Refutations*. London: Routledge.

Porter, R. (2003). *Blood and Guts: A Short History of Medicine*. London: Penguin Books.

Prainsack, B. (2016). Through Thick and Thin: Data Rich Medicine in the Era of Personalisation. In J. Vollman (Ed.), *The Ethics of Personalised Medicine: Critical Perspectives* (pp. 161–175). London: Routledge.

Price, D. (2009). *Human Tissue in Transplantation and Research*. Cambridge: Cambridge University Press.

Pykett, J. (2016). From Global Economic Change to Neuromolecular Capitalism. In J. De Vos & E. Pluth (Eds.), *Neuroscience and Critique: Exploring the Limits to the Neurological Turn* (pp. 81–99). London: Routledge.

Pykett, J. (2017). *Brain Culture: Shaping Policy through Neuroscience*. Bristol: Policy Press.

Racine, E., Bar-Ilan, O., & Illes, J. (2005). fMRI in the Public Eye. *Nature Reviews: Neuroscience, 6*(2), 159–164.

Rafi, I., Crinson, I., Dawes, M., Rafi, D., Pirmohamed, M., & Walter, F. M. (2020). The Implementation of Pharmacogenomics into UK General Practice: A Qualitative Study Exploring Barriers, Challenges and Opportunities. *Journal of Community Genetics, 11*(3), 269–277.

Rajagopalan, R., Nelson, A., & Fujimura, J. (2017). Race and Science in the Twenty-First Century. In U. Felt, R. Fouché, C. Miller, & L. Smith-Doerr (Eds.), *The Handbook of Science and Technology Studies* (4th ed., pp. 349–378). London, England: MIT Press.

Rajan, K. S. (2006). *Biocapital: The Constitution of Postgenomic Life*. Durham & London: Duke University Press.

Regalado, A. (1999). Inventing the Pharmacogenomics Business. *American Journal of Health System Pharma, 56*, 40–50.

Rehkopf, D., & Needham, B. (2019). The Impact of Race and Ethnicity in the Social Epigenomic Regulation of Disease. *Nutritional Epigenetics, 14*, 51–65.

Reichow, B., & Volkmar, F. (2018). Narrowing of 'Autism' in DSM-5 Runs Counter to Idea of Broad Spectrum. *Spectrum*, 9 May 2018.

Research England. (2020). Annual Funding Allocations 2019–20. Retrieved January 2020, from https://re.ukri.org/finance/annual-funding-allocations/annual-funding-allocations-2019-20/.

Rippon, G. (2019). *The Gendered Brain*. London: The Bodley Head.

Roberts, M., Kennedy, A., Chambers, D., & Khoury, M. (2017). The Current State of Implementation Science in Genomic Medicine: Opportunities for Improvement. *Genetics in Medicine, 19*(8), 858–863.

Roden, D., MacLeod, H., Relling, M., Mensah, G., Peterson, J., & Van Driest, S. (2019). Genomics Medicine 2—Pharmacogenomics. *The Lancet, 394*(10197), 521–532.

Rose, S. (1986). *Molecules and Minds: Essays on Biology and the Social Order*. Buckingham: Open University Press.

Rose, G. (1992). *The Strategy of Preventive Medicine*. Oxford: Oxford University Press.

Rose, N. (2007). *The Politics of Life Itself: Biomedicine, Power, and Subjectivity in the Twenty-First Century*. Oxford: Princeton University Press.

Rose, N. (2013). The Human Sciences in a Biological Age. *Theory, Culture, and Society, 30*(1), 3–34.

Rose, S. (2019, July 18). Pissing in the Snow. *London Review of Books, 41*(14).

Rose, N., & Abi-Rached, J. (2013). *Neuro: The New Brain Sciences and the Management of the Mind*. Princeton, NJ: Princeton University Press.

Rose, H., & Rose, S. (2012). *Genes, Cells and Brains: The Promethean Promises of the New Biology*. London: Verso.

Ross, S., Anand, S., Joseph, P., & Pare, G. (2012). Promises and Challenges of Pharmacogenetics: An Overview of Study Design, Methodological and Statistical Issues. *JRSM Cardiovascular Disease, 1*, 12.

Royal Pharmaceutical Society. (2014). New Medicines, Better Medicines, Better Use of Medicines. Retrieved from http://www.rpharms.com/promoting-pharmacy-pdfs/nmbmbu%2D%2D-full-report.pdf.

Ryan, L. (2012). 'You Must Be Very Intelligent…?': Gender and Science Subject Uptake. *International Journal of Gender, Science and Technology, 4*(2), 167–190.

Ryan, K., Loeppky, J., & Kilgore, D. (2009). A Forgotten Moment in Physiology: The Lovelace Women in Space Programme. *Advances in Physiology Education, 33*(3), 157–164.

Rylance, R. (2015). Grant Funders to Focus on Interdisciplinarity. Comment. *Nature, 525*, 313–315.

Sahakian, B., & Gottwald, J. (2017a). *Sex, Lies, and Brain Scans: How fMRI Reveals What Really Goes on in Our Minds*. Oxford: Oxford University Press.

Sahakian, B., & Gottwald, J. (2017b). *Sex, Lies, and Brain Scans: How fMRI Reveals What Really Goes on in Our Minds*. Oxford: Oxford University Press.

Salter, B., & Salter, C. (2017). Controlling New Knowledge: Genomic Science, Governance and The Politics of Bioinformatics. *Social Studies of Science, 47*(2), 263–287.

Sampson, A. (2017). *The Assemblage Brain: Sense Making in Neuroculture*. Minneapolis: University of Minnesota Press.

Sankey, H. (2009). Scientific Realism and the Semantic Incommensurability Thesis. *Studies in the History and Philosophy of Science, 40*(2), 196–202.

Sattler, S., Sauer, C., Mehlkop, G., & Graeff, P. (2013). The Rationale for Consuming Cognitive Enhancement Drugs in University Students and Teachers. *PLOS ONE, 8*(7), e68821.

Sayer, A. (1997). Essentialism, Social Constructionism, and Beyond. *The Sociological Review, 45*(3), 453–487.

Segerstråle, U. (2000). Science and Science Studies: Enemies or Allies? In U. Segerstråle (Ed.), *Beyond the Science Wars* (pp. 1–34). New York: State University of New York Press.

SES—Stanford Encyclopedia of Philosophy. (n.d.). *Einstein's Philosophy of Science*. Retrieved September 2019, from https://plato.stanford.edu/entries/einstein-philscience/.

Simmel, G. (1990). *The Philosophy of Money*. London: Routledge.

Simons, R., & Klopack, E. (2015). 'The Times They Are A-Changin' Gene Expression, Neuroplasticity, and Developmental Research. *Journal of Youth and Adolescence, 44*, 573–580.

Sismondo, S. (2010). *An Introduction to Science and Technology Studies* (2nd ed.). Chichester: Wiley-Blackwell.

Skinner, N., Lumey, L., Fleming, T., Sapienza, C., Hoyo, C., Aronica, L., et al. (2019). RW-2018—Research Workshop: The Effect of Nutrition on Epigenetic Status, Growth, and Health. *Journal of Parenteral and Enteral Nutrition, 43*(5), 627–637.

Slaby, J., & Choudhury, S. (2012). Proposal for a Critical Neuroscience. In S. Choudhury & J. Slaby (Eds.), *Critical Neuroscience: A Handbook of Social and Cultural Contexts of Neuroscience* (pp. 29–51). Chichester: Wiley Blackwell.

Slaby, J., & Choudhury, S. (2012). Introduction: Critical Neuroscience—Between Lifeworld and Laboratory. In S. Choudhury & J. Slaby (Eds.), *Critical Neuroscience: A Handbook of Social and Cultural Contexts of Neuroscience* (pp. 1–26). Chichester: Wiley Blackwell.

Smit, H., & Hacker, S. (2014). Seven Misconceptions About the Mereological Fallacy: A Compilation for the Perplexed. *Erkenntis, 79*, 1077–1097.

Smith, J., Zhao, W., Wang, X., Ratliff, S., Mukherjee, B., Kardia, S., et al. (2017). Neighborhood Characteristics Influence DNA Methylation of Genes Involved in Stress Response and Inflammation: The Multi-Ethnic Study of Atherosclerosis. *Epigenetics, 12*(8), 662–673.

Song, M., et al. (2015). Racial Differences in Genome-Wide Methylation Profiling and Gene Expression in Breast Tissues from Healthy Women. *Epigenetics, 10*(12), 1177–1187.

Sorell, T. (1991). *Scientism: Philosophy and the Infatuation with Science*. New York: Routledge.

Spear, B., et al. (2001). Clinical Application of Pharmacogenetics. *Trends in Molecular Medicine, 7*, 201–204.

Steinsbekk, K., Ursin, L., Skolbekkan, J., & Solberg, B. (2013). We're Not in it for the Money—Lay People's Moral Institutions on Commercial Use of 'Their' Biobank. *Medical Health Care and Philosophy, 16*, 151–162.

Straker, D. (2010). Changing Minds. Retrieved July 2019, from http://changingminds.org/.

Strech, D. (2015). Ethical Review of Biobank Research: Should REC's Review Each Release of Material from Biobanks Operating under an Already Approved Broad Consent and Data Protection Model? *European Journal of Medical Genetics, 58*, 545–549.

Sun, S., Lin, D., & Operario, D. (2020). Need for a Population Health Approach to Understand and Address Psychosocial Consequences of COVID-19. *Psychological Trauma: Theory, Research, Practice, and Policy, 12*(S1), S25–S27.

Synofzik, M. (2009). Ethically Justified, Clinically Applicable Criteria for Physician Decision-Making in Psychopharmacological Enhancement. *Neuroethics, 2*(2), 89–102.

Tallis, R. (2008). The Limitations of a Neurological Approach to Art. *Lancet, 372*, 19–20.

Tannock, I., & Hickman, J. (2016). Limits to Personalised Cancer Medicine. *New England Journal of Medicine, 375*(13), 1289–1294.

Temperton, J. (2016). Inside Sellafield: How the UK's Most Dangerous Nuclear Site Is Cleaning Up Its Act. *Wired*, 17 September 2016.

Thaler, R., & Sunstein, C. (2008). *Nudge: Improving Decisions About Health, Wealth and Happiness*. London: Yale University Press.

Thorén, H., & Persson, J. (2013). The Philosophy of Interdisciplinarity: Sustainability Science and Problem-Feeding. *Journal for General Philosophy of Science, 44*(2), 337–455.

Thornton, J. (2011). Neuroscience, Affect, and the Entrepreneurialization of Motherhood. *Communication and Critical/Cultural Studies, 8*(4), 399–424.

Titmuss, R. (1970). *The Gift Relationship: From Human Blood to Social Policy*. Bristol: Policy Press.

Tsuji, S. (2013). The Neurogenomics View of Neurological Diseases. *JAMA Neurology, 70*(6), 689–694.

Turner, A., Dallaire-Fortier, C., & Murtagh, M. (2013). Biobank Economics and the Commercialization Problem. *Spontaneous Generations, 7*(1), 69–80.

Tutton, R. (2014). *Genomics and the Reimagining of Personalized Medicine*. Farnham: Ashgate.

Tutton, R. (2016). Personal Genomics and Its Sociotechnical Transformations. In D. Kumar & R. Chadwick (Eds.), *Genomics and Society* (pp. 1–20). London: Academic Press.

UK Biobank. (2003). *Summary of the UK Biobank Consultation on the Ethics & Governance Framework*. Retrieved from www.ukbiobank.ac.uk/wp-content/uploads/2011/07/Summary-EGF-consultation.pdf?phpMyAdmin=trmKQlYdjjnQIgJ%2CfAzikMhEnx6.

UK Biobank. (2019). *About UK Biobank*. Retrieved January 2020, from https://www.ukbiobank.ac.uk/about-biobank-uk/.

UK Clinical Research Collaboration—UKCRC. (2015). *UK Health Research Analysis 2014*. London: UKCRC.

UK Research and Innovation—UKRI. (2019). *Annual Report and Accounts 2018–19*. HC207. Swindon: UKRI.

Ungar, S. (2016). Is This One It? Viral Moral Panics. In C. Krinsky (Ed.), *The Ashgate Research Companion to Moral Panics* (pp. 349–366). London: Routledge.

United Nations. (1997). *Gender Mainstreaming*. New York: Division for the Advancement of Women. United Nations Department for Economic and Social Affairs.

Universitetskanslersämbetet. (2018). *Universitet och högskolor. Årsrapport 2018*. Stockholm, SE: Universitetskanslersämbetet.

Van Noorden, R. (2015a). Interdisciplinary Research by the Numbers. *Nature, 525*(7569).

Van Noorden, R. (2015b). Interdisciplinary Research by the Numbers. *Nature, 525*, 306–307.

Walby, S. (1989). Theorising Patriarchy. *Sociology, 23*(2), 213–234.

Wastell, D., & White, S. (2017). *Blinded by Science: The Social Implications of Epigenetics and Neuroscience*. Bristol: Policy Press.

Watson, G. (2003). The Cognitive Revolution: A Historical Perspective. *Trends in Cognitive Sciences, 7*(3), 141–144.

Weinburg, S. (1992). *Dreams of a Final Theory: The Search for The Fundamental Laws of Nature*. New York: Random House.

Wellcome Trust. (2018). Wellcome Global Monitor 2018. Retrieved January 2020, from https://wellcome.ac.uk/reports/wellcome-global-monitor/2018.

Wikenius, E., Moe, V., Smith, L., Heiervang, E., & Berglund, A. (2019). DNA Methylation Changes in Infants between 6 and 52 Weeks. *Scientific Reports, 9*, 17587.

Winch, P. (1990). *The Idea of Social Science and Its Relation to Philosophy* (2nd ed.). London: Routledge.

Winecoff, A., & Huettel, S. (2017). Cognitive Control and Neuroeconomics. In T. Egner (Ed.), *The Wiley Handbook of Cognitive Control* (pp. 408–421). Chichester: John Wiley & Sons Ltd.

Women in Science (WISE). (n.d.). Retrieved January 2020, from https://www.wisecampaign.org.uk/resources/tag/statistics.

Woolgar, S. (2014). Struggles with Representation: Could It Be Otherwise? In C. Coopmans, J. Vertesi, M. Lynch, & S. Woolgar (Eds.), *Representation in Scientific Practice Revisited* (pp. 319–322). Cambridge, MA: MIT Press.

World Health Organisation. (2016). *International Classification of Diseases (ICD-10)*. Retrieved from https://icd.who.int/browse10/2016/en.

World Health Organisation. (2020). HIV/Aids—Global Observatory Data. Retrieved from https://www.who.int/gho/hiv/en/.

van der Wouden, et al. (2017). Implementing Pharmacogenomics in Europe: Design and Implementation strategy of the Ubiquitous Pharmacogenomics Consortium. *Clinical Pharmacology and Therapeutics, 101*(3), 341–358.

Wright, J. (2013). Epigenetics: Reversible Tags. *Nature, 498*, S10–S11.

Xafis, V., Schaefer, G., Labude, M., Brassington, I., Ballingtyne, A., Lim, H., et al. (2019). An Ethics Framework for Big Data in Health and Research. *Asian Bioethics Review, 11*, 227–254.

Yearley, S. (2005). *Making Sense of Science*. London: Sage.

Zhang, F., et al. (2011). Significant Differences in Global Genomic DNA Methylation by Gender and Race/Ethnicity in Peripheral Blood. *Epigenetics, 6*(5), 623–629.

The manufacturer's authorised representative in the EU is Springer Nature Customer Service Centre GmbH, Europaplatz 3, 69115 Heidelberg, Germany. If you have any concerns regarding our products, please contact ProductSafety@springernature.com

Printed and bound by CPI Group (UK) Ltd, Croydon, CR0 4YY
30/09/2026
02225448-0005